"After I was diagnosed with prostate cancer in 2001, the practical, sensitive and caring advice of Leah Jamnicky and her team made a world of difference in my treatment and recovery. They have now made their wise and valued insights available to everyone."

—**Allan Rock**, President and Vice-Chancellor of the University of Ottawa; former Canadian Minister of Justice, Canadian Minister of Health and Canada's ambassador to the United Nations

"The medical explanations, options presented and reassurances given combine in this book to alleviate the fear, uncertainty and anxiety we all face when staring at prostate cancer."

—**J. Barry Turner**, Director of Government Relations (Ottawa), Ducks Unlimited Canada; former Federal MP

"As a gay man, I wish this book had been around when I was first diagnosed with prostate cancer. No need to suffer in silence anymore—this medical team has written the definitive book on prostate cancer for all men, straight or gay."

—**Pearse Murray**, Radio Host, 103.9 Proud FM

"For the targeted audience of patients and their partners, this book hits the mark and I believe will prove to be extremely helpful in alleviating much of the fear of the unknown that comes with a diagnosis of prostate cancer. As such, I would recommend this book to friends, family, and patients."

—*B.C. Medical Journal*

THE CANADIAN GUIDE TO

PROSTATE CANCER

The Canadian Guide To

PROSTATE CANCER

Second Edition

Leah Jamnicky, RN
Robert Nam, MD, FRCSC
Editor: Helen Leask, PhD

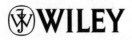

John Wiley & Sons Canada, Ltd.

Copyright © 2013 by SCRIPT Medical Press Inc.

All rights reserved. No part of this work covered by the copyright herein may be reproduced or used in any form or by any means—graphic, electronic or mechanical—without the prior written permission of the publisher. Any request for photocopying, recording, taping or placing in information storage and retrieval systems of any part of this book shall be directed in writing to The Canadian Copyright Licensing Agency (Access Copyright). For an Access Copyright license, visit www.access-copyright.ca or call toll-free 1-800-893-5777. For more information about Wiley products visit www.wiley.com.

Care has been taken to trace ownership of copyright material contained in this book. The publisher will gladly receive any information that will enable the correction of any reference or credit line in subsequent editions.

This publication contains the opinions and ideas of its authors and is designed to provide useful advice in regard to the subject matter covered. The authors and publisher are not engaged in rendering medical, therapeutic or other services in this publication. This publication is not intended to provide a basis for action in particular circumstances without consideration by a competent professional. The authors and publisher expressly disclaim any responsibility for any liability, loss or risk, personal or otherwise, which is incurred as a consequence, directly or indirectly, of the use and application of any of the contents of this book.

Library and Archives Canada Cataloguing in Publication Data
Jamnicky, Leah, 1963-
    The Canadian guide to prostate cancer / Leah Jamnicky, Robert Nam; editor, Helen Leask. — 2nd ed.

Includes bibliographical references and index.
Issued also in electronic formats.
ISBN 978-1-118-36283-9

    1. Prostate—Cancer—Popular works. 2. Prostate—Surgery—Popular works.
I. Nam, Robert, 1970- II. Leask, Helen III. Title. IV. Title: Prostate cancer.

RD587.J34 2012   616.99'463   C2012-905321-X

Publishing Credits
Editorial team for 1st Edition: Dennis Jeanes, Jenny Lass, Sarah von Riedemann, Jaime Woo
Editorial management for 2nd Edition: Pinay Kainth
Book illustrations: Zane Waldman
Author photographs: Mariko Yaguchi-Chow, Doug Nicholson (Media Source), Robert Linowski

Production Credits
Book design: Angela Bobotsis
Cover design 1st Edition: Mike Chan, David McFee
Cover design 2nd Edition: Adrian So
Typesetter: Laserwords
Printer: Friesens
Image on page © 2008 Sunnybrook Health Sciences Centre.

Photograph on page 123 courtesy of Doug Nicholson/MediaSource.
Poem on page 174 republished with permission of Shambhala Publications Inc, from *The Erotic Spirit: An Anthology of Poems of Sensuality, Love and Longing*, edited by Sam Hamill, © 1999; permission conveyed through Copyright Clearance Center, Inc.

John Wiley & Sons Canada, Ltd.
6045 Freemont Blvd.
Mississauga, Ontario
L5R 4J3

Printed in Canada

1 2 3 4 5 FP 17 16 15 14 13

In memory of my father, the Rev Paul Jamnicky,
who always said, "be all that you can be."
To my loving family who are always
there to support me in all that I do:
my mother, Betty, my sisters, Lydia and Rachael,
my brother, Paul, and their wonderful spouses,
Brent, Randy and Jamie; my amazing nephew,
Ryan, and my beautiful nieces, Nicky,
Ally, Sophie and Cady.

L.J.

To my loving wife, Yuna, and my children,
Matthew and Amy.

R.N.

To my father, the late Michael John McAllister Leask:
Oxford emeritus fellow and enthusiast for life.

H.L.

contents

The inside story on prostate cancer surgery ∿ What if treatment doesn't work? ∿ Pros and cons of other cancer options

acknowledgements

This book would not have been possible without the support of my family, friends and colleagues, who are always there for me offering their support and encouragement. They helped me to make this book a reality. Thank you to my mentors, Dr John Trachtenberg, Dr Neil Fleshner, Dr Michael Jewett, Dr Michael Robinette and Dr Tony Finelli. Particular thanks are due to Dr Andrew Matthew, Valerie Marshall BSP, April Guthrie RN, Lisa Andrews RN, Kristen Currie MA, Daniel Santa Mina BSc CEP, Kateri Corr RN, Catherine Rowland RN, Mariko Yaguchi-Chow, Rachael Brassard BSc, Lydia Bartell RN, Lucia Evans RN, Chrisa Goebel RN, Judy Costello RN, Silvie Crawford RN, Gail James, Dr Rob Bristow, Dr Alex Zlotta, Dr Girish Kulkarni and Michael Nesbitt. I am extremely grateful to the prostate cancer survivor volunteers who so generously give of themselves to help others diagnosed with prostate cancer; I marvel at their dedication and passion for life, which continues to inspire me.

—Leah Jamnicky

I would like to thank and acknowledge all my patients who underwent surgery for prostate cancer, whose experiences have made this book possible. I would also like to thank Dr Andrew Loblaw, radiation oncologist, at Sunnybrook Health Sciences Centre for his comments. Finally, many thanks to the Canadian Cancer Society, Prostate Cancer Canada and

the Canadian Institute for Health Research (CIHR) for their
ongoing support for my research.

—Robert Nam

Specialized but essential books need an army of believers
to make them a reality in Canada, and The Canadian Guide
to Prostate Cancer is no exception. Robert Harris, Angela
Bobotsis, Jenny Lass, Leah Fairbank, Dennis Jeanes, Malcolm
Lester, Gerry Jenkison, Martha Peacock and Dave McFee are
especially worthy of mention for the skills and enthusiasm that
made both editions of *Prostate* possible. I am grateful to Nancy
Richardson and all at SCRIPT for their unflagging patience
when our books take over normal life. I would also like to thank
the patients who shared their experiences with me and gave
the cold facts a beating heart. Finally, Liz Leask, Donald Leask,
Stuart Leask, Ali Leask, Kate Gordon, Martha Byrt, Milo
Leask and Tony Plut keep my "campfire of fortune" burning.
Thank you.

—Helen Leask

disclaimer

The information provided in this book may not apply to all patients, all clinical situations, all hospitals or all eventualities, and is not intended to be a substitute for the advice of a qualified physician or other medical professional. Always consult a qualified physician about anything that affects your health, especially before starting an exercise program or any therapy not prescribed by your doctor.

While the authors made every reasonable effort to include the most current data and practices in this publication, it is not intended to be an exhaustive review of the scientific literature and it should not be read as such.

The naming of any organization, product, or therapy in this book does not imply endorsement by the authors or publisher, and the omission of any such names does not indicate disapproval by the authors or publisher.

The views in this book do not necessarily reflect those of Prostate Cancer Canada.

introduction

I If you or a loved one is facing prostate cancer, we hope our book will bring you some peace of mind. Our goal is to help you better understand your options so that you can make informed treatment decisions and feel in control of what happens next.

The reality is that prostate cancer is, for most men, a very slow-growing cancer. You will probably have plenty of time to make up your mind about how to face this new challenge in your life. Whatever you eventually decide, we are with you all the way.

First, we'll outline the basics on prostate cancer. Chapter 1 covers prostate anatomy and the differences between benign (non-cancerous) and malignant (cancerous) prostate disease. If you are reading this book to find out if you can avoid prostate cancer or detect it early, Chapters 2 and 3 are for you. We hear a lot of non-scientific theories about how to prevent prostate cancer, so Chapter 2 takes a good, hard look at the real science and what we *do* know. The good news is that some types of prostate cancer can be prevented by a healthy lifestyle. Prostate cancer screening is also important because it can pick up prostate cancer in its earliest stages. Chapter 3 looks at all the tests for prostate cancer, including the controversial PSA test, so that you can fully understand what these tests could mean for you. If your tests show that your prostate problems are non-cancerous, Chapter 4 gives you the complete rundown on benign prostatic hyperplasia (BPH).

If you have been diagnosed with prostate cancer, it's important to understand the pros and cons of surgery versus other treatment options, including doing nothing at all ("watchful waiting") (Chapter 5). If you and your physician decide that surgery is your best option, our book will give you a step-by-step description of what to expect before, during and after your operation, including tips for more effective healing, pain management and lifestyle changes (Chapters 6 to 12).

Most men reading this book will be concerned about how prostate cancer might affect their sex lives. Chapter 13 covers everything you need to know about sex after prostate cancer, in clear, unambiguous language. The encouraging news is that there is no anatomical reason why prostate cancer treatment will affect your libido or your ability to enjoy sex, and this chapter tells you why. Recovering from any serious illness can be hard and one of the most miraculous medicines of all is simple exercise. Even if you have never really exercised before, Chapter 14 will walk you through some simple steps you can take to feel better fast. Chapter 15 offers gay Canadian men information on prostate cancer, tailored to their needs.

The book also includes a glossary, a summary of medications, a "Who's Who" of hospital staff, a list of valuable resources and a personal diary where you can write down your medical history, important contact information, appointment dates, medications and symptoms.

Although the wealth of detail we've provided may seem a bit overwhelming, arming yourself with this information will help you become an active participant in managing your disease and help you regain control of your long-term well-being. Above all, we encourage you to be positive.

Good luck!

Chapter 1

prostate cancer and you

What Happens in This Chapter
- Overview of prostate disease
- Anatomy of the urinary system and prostate gland
- The facts on prostate cancer
- Who is at greatest risk for prostate cancer?

The prostate gland has several functions. As well as producing fluids that nourish sperm, it acts as a urinary sphincter and its muscles help semen flow during ejaculation. That's why the prostate is strategically located just below the bladder and surrounds the upper part of the urethra, the tube from which you urinate and ejaculate. Prostate cancer is the commonest type of cancer in men and the third leading cause of cancer death. It is important to diagnose prostate cancer at an early stage where there is only a small amount of cancer and it is confined to the prostate gland. The earlier the cancer is detected, the higher your chances of being cured. There are many treatment options for patients with prostate cancer that is detected early, including surgery and radiation. These procedures aim to maximize cancer control while preserving your quality of life.

The Facts About Prostate Disease

There are three kinds of prostate disorder: inflammation of the prostate gland (**prostatitis**), benign prostate enlargement, or **benign prostatic hyperplasia** (**BPH**), and prostate cancer. All three conditions are common, with prostate cancer and BPH being more common in men aged 50 and older. Although these disorders can share many of the same symptoms, they all have different causes and treatments.

Prostatitis occurs most often in young and middle-aged men but can occur at any age. The symptoms are severe pain in areas around the prostate (called pelvic pain) and sometimes back pain. Urination may be more frequent than usual and cause a "burning" pain. Prostatitis can be a difficult problem to fix because we do not know a lot about what causes it or what consequences it might have.

Normally, treatment is with a long course of antibiotics—usually for 4 to 6 weeks. Other medications include anti-inflammatories to help reduce inflammation and pain. Sometimes medications used to treat BPH help, but there are no surgical treatments for prostatitis.

Prostatitis can be a very frustrating disease for both the patient and physician. The treatments do not always work, and men are often forced to live with their symptoms, which can severely affect their quality of life. Further research is certainly needed to improve this situation. This book will not be talking about prostatitis in detail, so please consult your doctor if you need further information.

The older you get, the more likely you are to have an enlarged prostate, or BPH. Only 8 percent of men aged 30 to 40 have enlarged prostates—compared to 50 percent of men aged 50 to 60, and 90 percent of men aged 80 or more.

However, an enlarged prostate is not an immediate ticket to the operating room. BPH is almost considered a normal part of aging. Importantly, BPH is completely different from prostate cancer, and if you have BPH it does not automatically mean that you will develop prostate cancer. The improved treatment options available to men with BPH today mean that only about 1 in 20 patients need surgery—those with the most severe clinical symptoms or who develop medical problems from the condition. BPH can be effectively treated with medication that shrinks and relaxes the tissues of the prostate gland. For more on BPH and how it is treated, see Chapter 4.

Even if you have prostate cancer, there is reassuring news. Although prostate cancer affects 1 in 7 men during their lifetime, it is being caught more frequently and earlier as a result of improved awareness and new screening procedures introduced in the late 1980s. With current treatment methods, most men with localized disease can be cured.

Prostate Anatomy and Function

The prostate is a good example of evolution's economy of design, making do with one set of plumbing instead of creating two. However, this piggybacking of the reproductive system onto the urinary system creates problems that most often appear at a time in a man's life when he might be happier passing urine in a strong, steady stream than passing on his DNA.

The Urinary Journey
Urine is filtered from the blood by the kidneys and then runs into the **bladder** through two tubes, called the **ureters** (see Figure 1–1).

Figure 1-1 The Urinary Journey

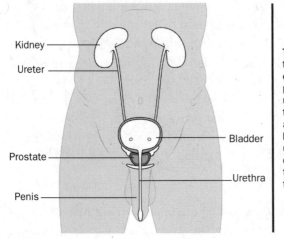

Kidney

Ureter

Prostate

Penis

Bladder

Urethra

The kidneys filter the blood and eliminate waste products such as urine. The urine flows through the ureters and collects in the bladder. When you urinate, the bladder contracts to push the urine out through the urethra.

The bladder consists of a balloon-like membrane surrounded by layers of smooth-muscle tissue, collectively called the **detrusor**. When you urinate, nerve pathways signal the detrusor to contract. After you empty your bladder, your brain signals the detrusor muscle to relax. Much of the conscious control you have over urination is from learning as a child to inhibit spontaneous contractions of your bladder.

The bladder is an amazing organ that can expand to hold about half a litre (16 oz) of urine before you have a conscious sensation of fullness. You produce up to 1.5 litres (48 oz) of urine every 24 hours. Rings of muscle (called the **internal sphincter**) at the bottom of the bladder and prostate gland form a neck that can open up or clamp shut.

Urine leaves the bladder through a tube called the urethra and exits through the penis. You control the flow of urine with a donut-shaped muscle called the **external sphincter**, which acts as a stop valve when contracted.

How Do You Urinate?

When you decide to urinate, the bladder contracts, the internal sphincter of the bladder's neck relaxes, and urine flows into the urethra. When you consciously relax the external sphincter, urine passes out.

What Is Semen? [**MORE DETAIL**]

Semen is made up of sperm and a lubricating, nourishing fluid called seminal fluid. Most of the seminal fluid is produced by the seminal vesicles. The rest is made by other organs, including the prostate.

The Urethra–Prostate Connection

In addition to emptying the bladder, the urethra serves as the passageway for ejaculating sperm. Thin tubes called the **vas deferens** loop back from each testicle for about 46 cm (18 inches) along both sides of the bladder (see Figure 1–2). These tubes transport sperm with a rippling, muscular motion. Also entering from each side are ducts from the **seminal vesicles**, tubular structures tucked up underneath the bladder. The vas deferens and the seminal vesicles meet, then merge with the urethra.

So where does the prostate fit into all of this? Although we call it the prostate "gland," the prostate is actually a collection of glands and smooth-muscle fibres encased in a fibrous, muscular capsule. The prostate sits across the upper urethra, the vas deferens and the ducts of the seminal vesicles, just between the neck of the bladder and the external sphincter (see Figure 1–2).

Figure 1-2 The Urethra–Prostate Connection

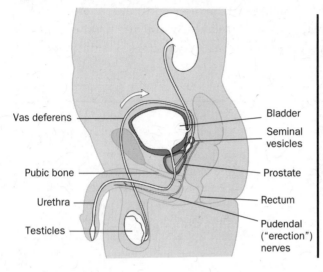

Vas deferens

Pubic bone

Urethra

Testicles

Bladder

Seminal vesicles

Prostate

Rectum

Pudendal ("erection") nerves

Sperm are produced by the testes, and then travel up though the vas deferens. The sperm mix with seminal fluids from the prostate and other glands to form semen, which leaves the body through the urethra during ejaculation.

The prostate consists of an inner zone (called the **transition zone**) and an outer (or **peripheral**) zone, and is also divided into right and left sides, called lobes. Prostate cancer usually arises from the peripheral zone, whereas BPH usually originates in the transition zone. The wide portion nearest the bladder is the **base**, and the tip farthest from the bladder is the **apex**. Just a few millimetres behind the prostate is the front wall of the rectum. Between them run networks of microscopic blood vessels and the all-important nerve pathways that are needed for erections.

At birth, the prostate is no bigger than a pea. At puberty, it grows rapidly, attaining its adult shape and size (about the size of a small walnut) at around age 20. During sexual activity, it secretes a thin, milky fluid that is pumped into the urethra through tiny ducts. Once there, the fluid mixes with the rest of the semen to make it flow more easily (see More Detail box on page 5).

Prostate Cancer

Compared with other forms of **cancer**, prostate tumours are slow growing. A **tumour** that is confined within the prostate gland may take 5 to 15 years to spread to other organs. Therefore, the younger you are, the more likely it is that you will be affected by the growth and spread of prostate cancer. Older men diagnosed with prostate cancer will likely die *with* the disease, while younger men are more likely to die *from* the disease, just because they have many more potential years to live.

Prostate cancer can be detected at any stage in its development and progression, depending on how often a man goes for a "wellness" check, what symptoms he is having, the location of the tumour and other factors. The cancer may be confined within the prostate gland (called **localized prostate cancer**), or it may have spread from the prostate gland throughout the body to organs such as the **lymph nodes**, bones, lungs and liver (called **metastatic prostate cancer**). Cancer is confined to the prostate in 9 out of 10 men diagnosed with prostate cancer, while it has already spread in the other 1 out of 10.

Early-stage prostate cancer generally doesn't cause noticeable symptoms because it occurs in the outer layer of the prostate gland and does not interfere with urination (see Figure 1–3).

Despite the fact that there are no symptoms, the reason that many men with prostate cancer are diagnosed in the early stages is because of the widespread use of a blood test called **prostate specific antigen** (**PSA**). This blood test was introduced in 1987. It can detect the presence of prostate cancer early on and has revolutionized how prostate cancer is diagnosed and treated. For more on PSA testing, see pages 30–34.

When the tumour has increased in size, it can cause symptoms similar to benign prostate enlargement. Back pain and bone pain may mean that the cancer has spread to other parts of the body, such as the spine and pelvis.

Who Is Most Likely to Get Prostate Cancer?

Some men have a much greater chance of getting prostate cancer than others. Scientists have spent years trying to figure out the list of prostate cancer risk factors in an effort to predict (and protect) those men most likely to get this form of cancer.

The first and most important risk factor for prostate cancer is age. So much so, that prostate cancer should really be considered a disease of aging since the older you get, the more likely it is that you will get prostate cancer. In particular, the risk shoots up when you turn 50 years old, which is why experts recommend that you see your physician regularly for testing after age 50.

Another risk factor is your ethnic background. Men of African ancestry are more likely to develop prostate cancer than Caucasian men. Asians have the lowest risk. The reason for these differences is still unknown, although it is likely to be a combination of heredity and "environmental" factors such as diet. The reason we know it is not purely down to genes is that Asian countries such as China, Japan and Korea have much lower rates of prostate cancer than Western countries. However, when Asians immigrate to North America, their risk for prostate cancer starts to increase to the level seen among Caucasians. Thus, dietary and environmental factors unique to each country and culture may play a big part in triggering the development of prostate cancer. This is good news, as it suggests prostate cancer may be preventable in many men. This is explored in more detail in Chapter 2.

Genetics do matter though, because the third biggest risk factor for prostate cancer is having a relative with the disease. If your father, brother, uncle, grandfather or any member of your blood-related family has prostate cancer, you are at least twice as likely to get it yourself. The more male relatives you have with prostate cancer, the greater your own risk— up to an 8-fold increase. Some families have what is known as "hereditary prostate cancer," in

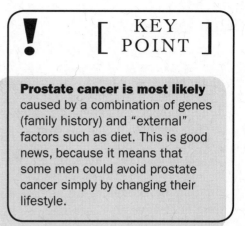

! [KEY POINT]

Prostate cancer is most likely caused by a combination of genes (family history) and "external" factors such as diet. This is good news, because it means that some men could avoid prostate cancer simply by changing their lifestyle.

which many members of the same family, sometimes three successive generations, develop prostate cancer at a young age (under 55). If you do have a family history of prostate cancer, your physician may recommend that you start screening tests earlier than age 50, for example when you turn 40 years of age. For more on the genetics of prostate cancer, see More Detail box on next page.

Figure 1-3 Prostate Cancer

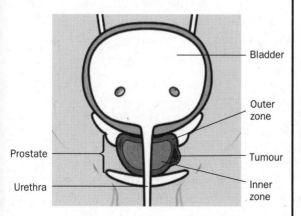

Bladder

Outer zone

Prostate

Tumour

Urethra

Inner zone

There are usually few symptoms in the early stages of prostate cancer because the tumour tends to grow slowly in the outer zone of the prostate, away from the urethra. In later stages, the tumour may grow large enough to squeeze the urethra or other structures.

Do You Have Prostate
Cancer in Your Genes?

[MORE
DETAIL]

Prostate cancer seems to run in families, so many studies have tried to find a "prostate cancer gene." Several genes appear to be linked with prostate cancer, although how they cause trouble is still unclear. The most heavily studied is a gene defect located on chromosome 1 called the hereditary prostate cancer-1 (*HPC1*) gene. Another gene generating a lot of excitement in scientific circles is located on chromosome 8. However, more scientific research is needed before we have a genetic test to help diagnose prostate cancer.

Apart from these major risk factors, other features of your life may stack the prostate cancer odds against you, such as obesity, and eating too much fat and red meat. These are covered in more detail in Chapter 2.

Finally, it is worth taking a look at what is *not* linked to prostate cancer. Vasectomy — a permanent method of birth control for men — came under fire in the past for "causing" prostate cancer. However, scientific studies have not confirmed this, and most experts do not believe there is a connection between the two. Similarly, whatever other terrible things smoking does to your health, it does not appear to be linked to prostate cancer.

What Happens Next?

If your doctor suspects that you have prostate cancer, or just wants to rule it out, he or she will order some tests, described in Chapter 3. Early detection of your prostate cancer can give you a significant advantage because the cancer is easier to cure at this early stage, and many treatment options are still open to you.

Chapter 2

is prostate cancer preventable?

What Happens in This Chapter
- Talking to your doctor
- The links between diet and prostate cancer
- The links between obesity and prostate cancer
- Prescription medication to prevent prostate cancer

Perhaps one of the most common questions men ask is, "Can I do anything to prevent prostate cancer?" The answer is an overwhelming "Yes!" Studies show that making lifestyle changes, such as eating the right foods and losing weight, may help prevent prostate cancer. There is even prescription medication that you can take as a form of prevention. But be sure to talk to your doctor about prostate cancer prevention options to make sure you are getting the best and safest treatment possible.

Talk to Your Doctor

There is a lot of information about prostate cancer prevention out there, and it can be difficult to figure out what is more helpful than harmful. You may already have discovered this when you Googled "prostate cancer prevention" and got tens of thousands of hits! Some of this information is backed up by scientific research and some is not; plus, many websites give wrong information. It is also important to remember that research is always evolving — generating new concepts, disproving old ones and improving on what we already know. This means that yesterday's recommendations are not necessarily today's, as we will see with the vitamin E, selenium and finasteride stories. That's why it's important to discuss prostate cancer prevention strategies with your physician or specialist. He or she can guide you through the sea of resources available on preventing prostate cancer and, more importantly, can help you determine which prevention strategies are right for you. As a starting point, this chapter will give you an overview of the science behind prostate cancer prevention so that you can have a productive discussion with your physician. You may also find it helpful to visit the US National Cancer Institute (http://www.cancer.gov/) and the Canadian Cancer Society Research Institute (http://www.cancer.ca) websites for reliable updated recommendations and information on new research.

Taking Alternatives?
Tell Your Doctor!

[MORE DETAIL]

In 2000, Dr Nam and his medical colleagues at the University of Toronto conducted a survey of 268 urology clinic patients with no history of prostate cancer. About 25 percent of these men were on some form of alternative therapy to prevent prostate cancer, and 24 percent of them had not told their physician about their self-treatments, some of which were potentially dangerous to their health! So be sure to discuss prostate cancer prevention strategies with your doctor before trying any preventive measures.

Diet and Prostate Cancer

Food can have a powerful effect on the body. Eating the wrong foods can make you sick, whereas eating the right foods can heal you or even prevent you from becoming ill in the first place. Not surprisingly, researchers have identified several foods and nutrients that may help to prevent prostate cancer, plus others that may actually promote the development of the disease. Although there are no guarantees when it comes to cancer prevention, this section will give you some guidance on what to eat and what not to eat to stack the odds in your favour.

Foods and Nutrients That May Prevent Prostate Cancer

Antioxidants

The top foods that have been associated with preventing prostate cancer are tomatoes and tomato products, cruciferous vegetables (such as broccoli and cauliflower), soy and legumes (such as peas, peanuts and beans). Researchers believe it is the antioxidant properties of these foods and nutrients that hold the key to their medicinal power. The **antioxidants** vitamin E and

13

selenium had also been linked to prostate cancer prevention, but this is no longer the case (see below).

An antioxidant is a chemical that reduces the damaging effects of oxygen by-products on tissues. Even though we need oxygen to provide energy for the individual cells in our body (we do this by breathing), processing oxygen within the body produces by-products that can potentially harm our cells. These by-products are called **free radicals** and **peroxides**, and they lead to what is known as **oxidative stress**. Fortunately, our cells are able to neutralize this stress with antioxidant proteins and quickly repair any cell damage, including damage to DNA.

However, this fine balance between the production and neutralization of oxidative stress can be upset for various reasons, particularly by external influences such as radiation, environmental pollutants, abnormal immune function or uncontrolled inflammation within the body. When our cells lose the ability to protect us from oxidative stress, we run the risk of developing diseases such as heart disease, neurological disorders (e.g., Alzheimer's disease) and many types of cancer. That's why it's important to boost your antioxidant levels by eating foods and nutrients with antioxidant properties that could help reduce the effects of oxidative stress and, in turn, reduce your risk of developing prostate cancer.

Lycopene

Lycopene is an antioxidant found in tomatoes and is responsible for their red colour. Although lycopene is found in other foods, such as watermelon, the main sources of this antioxidant in our westernized diet are tomatoes and tomato sauce. Many studies show that men who report that they eat a lot of tomatoes have a lower rate of prostate cancer than men who eat very few tomatoes and tomato products. Other studies have linked high blood lycopene levels to a lower risk of prostate cancer.

However, researchers have not identified how much tomato we need to eat to receive the most benefit from lycopene. Lycopene supplements are also available, but, again, there is no agreement on how many to take or how often to take them. Several studies suggest that 6 mg/day of lycopene may be beneficial, and it is easily obtained through our regular diet (see table).

Food/drink	Portion	Lycopene content (mg)
Vegetable juice cocktail	1 cup	23.4
Tomato juice	1 cup	22.0
Pasta sauce	½ cup	21.5
Watermelon	1 slice (about 285 g)	13.0
Stewed tomato	1 cup	10.3
Raw tomato	1 regular tomato	3.2
Ketchup	1 tbsp	2.5

Sulforaphane

Cruciferous vegetables, including broccoli, cauliflower, cabbage, brussels sprouts and bok choy, contain an antioxidant called sulforaphane. Unlike tomatoes, the ability of these foods to prevent prostate cancer has not been extensively studied. However, data suggest that eating at least 5 or more servings of cruciferous vegetables per week may reduce the risk of developing prostate cancer by 10 to 20 percent.

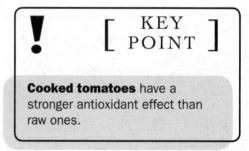

! [KEY POINT]

Cooked tomatoes have a stronger antioxidant effect than raw ones.

Isoflavones

Soy and legumes have also been shown to reduce the risk of prostate cancer. These foods are central to diets in Asia, where the rate of prostate cancer is the world's lowest. Studies have supported this observation by showing that men who have soy-based or legume-based diets have lower rates of prostate cancer than men who do not eat a lot of soy and legumes.

The beneficial effects of soy and legumes have been attributed to their high concentration of isoflavones, antioxidants that are part of the phytoestrogen family. Researchers have a theory that isoflavones may help protect men because phytoestrogens influence the production and use of hormones, such as estrogens and testosterone, that play an important role in prostate cancer. Laboratory studies confirm that phytoestrogens reduce the formation of prostate cancer cells in test tubes and inhibit their growth.

Asian Men and Prostate Cancer [MORE DETAIL]

Asian men have a much lower risk of developing prostate cancer than Caucasian men. However, when Asian men immigrate and adopt a westernized lifestyle, their rate of prostate cancer increases. One reason for this could be changes in diet.

Vitamin E and Selenium
The vitamin E and selenium story is a classic example of why researchers need to do the right medical studies to see if a particular substance could prevent prostate cancer. The primary nutrient once linked to prostate cancer prevention was vitamin E. This vitamin's protective antioxidant effect was discovered accidentally when a large US study examined whether taking vitamin E could prevent lung cancer. Although the study showed that vitamin E did not prevent lung cancer, it revealed

that prostate cancer among men who took vitamin E was 30 to 40 percent lower than for men who did not take it.

Selenium is a trace element in many foods, including grains, fish, meat, poultry, dairy products and eggs. Similar to vitamin E, selenium was found to be associated with low rates of prostate cancer quite by chance. Because of these studies, sales of vitamin E and selenium took off, and every prostate-friendly health supplement contained them.

However, scientists and doctors felt more research was needed in this area, so the US National Cancer Institute funded a large multimillion dollar study to test whether vitamin E and selenium could indeed prevent prostate cancer. The study was called SELECT and involved about 35,000 men in the US and Canada. Researchers used the approach preferred by the medical community for doing rigorous medical studies—a **randomized clinical trial**. The 35,000 men were randomly assigned to one of four groups and took vitamin E, selenium, both or a **placebo** (a sugar pill that essentially does nothing). As the study progressed, researchers began looking at the results, and what they found shocked the medical world. Men who took vitamin E alone actually developed higher rates of prostate cancer compared to men who did not. Men who took selenium alone had the same rate of prostate cancer as men who didn't take it, but, surprisingly, men taking selenium developed higher rates of diabetes. Based on these results, the study was terminated early. Thus, vitamin E and selenium should *not* be taken to prevent prostate cancer.

Green Tea and Red Wine

Two common drinks that may prevent prostate cancer are green tea and red wine. Studies in Asian countries, where green tea is popular, have shown that rates of prostate cancer are lower among men who drink a lot of green tea compared to those who give it a miss. Similarly, a study showed that regular red wine drinkers in North America had a 6 percent reduction in their risk of developing prostate cancer for every glass of red wine consumed. Before you run out and stock up on red wine, however, a word of caution: other studies have not found a relationship between red wine consumption and prostate cancer risk. More research is needed to understand how green tea and red wine could prevent prostate cancer—and whether they really do.

Fish

A high fish intake has also been suggested to reduce the risk of developing prostate cancer. The long-chain omega-3 fatty acids found in fish appear to slow the growth of cancer cells in the laboratory, but researchers don't know why. The rich vitamin D content of fish (see table in Self-Help box) may also be responsible for its cancer-protecting effects, since vitamin D may be protective.

Vitamin D

Although some comes from our diet (see Self-Help box), most vitamin D in our bodies is activated when we are exposed to sunlight. Thus, people who live in northern climates, who generally experience less sun exposure, tend to be vitamin D deficient. So why is all this relevant to prostate cancer?

Laboratory studies in test tubes and animals have shown that vitamin D halts the growth of prostate cancer cells. Also, people with low levels of vitamin D seem to have a higher rate of prostate cancer. These findings suggest that vitamin D may have a role in preventing prostate cancer cells from growing and spreading.

Studies have shown that men who live in northern climates do indeed have a higher rate of prostate cancer than their neighbours closer to the equator. Interestingly, elderly men, who generally get less sunlight because of inactivity, and men with dark skin, whose skin melanin blocks ultraviolet rays, are two of the highest risk groups for prostate cancer.

One explanation for these findings is that the less sunlight you get, the lower your vitamin D levels and the less "vitamin D protection" you get—although this has yet to be proved.

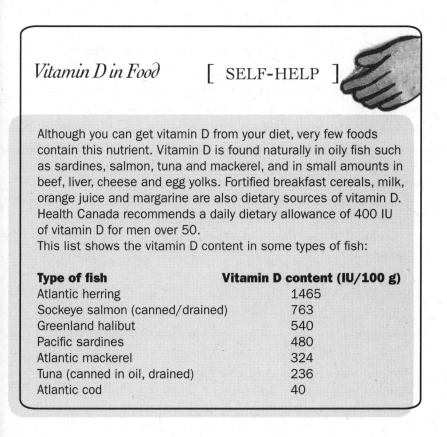

Vitamin D in Food   [SELF-HELP]

Although you can get vitamin D from your diet, very few foods contain this nutrient. Vitamin D is found naturally in oily fish such as sardines, salmon, tuna and mackerel, and in small amounts in beef, liver, cheese and egg yolks. Fortified breakfast cereals, milk, orange juice and margarine are also dietary sources of vitamin D. Health Canada recommends a daily dietary allowance of 400 IU of vitamin D for men over 50.
This list shows the vitamin D content in some types of fish:

Type of fish	Vitamin D content (IU/100 g)
Atlantic herring	1465
Sockeye salmon (canned/drained)	763
Greenland halibut	540
Pacific sardines	480
Atlantic mackerel	324
Tuna (canned in oil, drained)	236
Atlantic cod	40

Zinc

Zinc helps to maintain the human immune system and promote wound healing. Although there are very few studies that directly link zinc to prostate cancer prevention, laboratory studies have shown that zinc accumulates in the prostate, and this may inhibit prostate cancer cells from growing. Our body's requirement for zinc is very low and easily obtained through a well-balanced diet. The daily maximum intake of zinc is 40 mg, but zinc supplementation should not exceed 11 mg per day. Zinc is found in poultry, eggs, liver and seafood, particularly in oysters and crab meat.

Foods and Nutrients That May Cause Prostate Cancer

Red Meat and Saturated Fats

Two key foods that researchers believe may cause prostate cancer are red meat and saturated fats in general. Red meat is problematic for two reasons. The first is the actual content of the meat—many studies have linked meat protein and saturated fats to cancer formation. Large studies that followed the diets of men over many years found that heavy meat eaters and those who ate fat-rich foods had a significantly higher risk for developing prostate cancer. Meat protein and saturated fats may trigger cancer by affecting hormonal factors and oxidative stress (see page 13).

The other problem with red meat is that when it is grilled or barbecued, it produces chemicals called heterocyclic amines (HA), which the US Department of Health and Human Services added in 2005 to their list of substances that could reasonably cause cancer in humans. Animal studies seem to confirm that HAs cause prostate cancer, but the amount of HA used in these experiments was much higher than the amount humans normally consume.

However, it is also important to keep in mind that beef has many health benefits. It contains vitamins, and minerals such as zinc, that protect against prostate cancer development. So eliminating beef completely from your diet is not necessary.

Calcium

Although calcium is generally considered to be good for health, high amounts of this mineral have been associated with increased prostate cancer risk. One study found that men who drank large quantities of milk or consumed excessive amounts of calcium in food (more than 2000 mg per day) had a higher chance of developing prostate cancer. However, the reason for this is still unclear, and other studies have not reproduced the finding. It is important not to cut calcium from your diet. You should consume the recommended daily allowance of 1000 to 1200 mg. *Canada's Food Guide* recommends 2 to 3 servings of milk each day.

This is especially true for patients undergoing hormone treatments, since this type of therapy causes greater bone loss, which means a higher risk of wrist, hip and spine fractures. If you consider that osteoporosis is already a fairly common bone disease in older men without prostate cancer, you'll appreciate the benefit of calcium on bone health.

Prostate Cancer in Vegetarians [MORE DETAIL]

Even among vegetarians, such as the strictly vegetarian Seventh-Day Adventist religious group, the rate of prostate cancer is high, so eliminating meat from your diet will not necessarily prevent prostate cancer.

Help Yourself to Prevention

[SELF-HELP]

Here is a summary of foods and nutrients that may help prevent or increase the risk of prostate cancer. If you plan on taking supplements, talk to your physician about the right dose for you in view of any medical conditions you may have or drugs you may be taking.

Foods and nutrients to eat
- Tomatoes and tomato products
- Cruciferous vegetables
- Soy
- Legumes
- Green tea
- Red wine (in moderation)
- Fish
- Calcium
- Vitamin D
- Zinc

Foods and nutrients to limit
- Red meat
- Saturated fats
- Excessive calcium supplementation

Obesity and Prostate Cancer

The number of people who are obese in North America has increased dramatically since the 1980s, along with the many health problems associated with obesity. Obesity can contribute to the development of cardiovascular disease, diabetes, arthritis and, of course, cancers. In particular, many studies have consistently linked obesity to a high prostate cancer risk. Moreover, past studies have shown a lower rate of prostate cancer among Olympic athletes. This discrepancy may be related to hormonal imbalances caused by the excessive fat tissue in obese men.

Measuring Obesity With BMI [MORE DETAIL]

> One of the ways to measure obesity is with body mass index (BMI), which factors in your age, weight and height to produce a number that represents how healthy or unhealthy your weight is. If your BMI is 18.5 to 24.6, your weight is normal; if your score is 25 to 29.9, you are considered overweight; if your BMI is 30 or higher, you are considered obese.

Obesity may also affect PSA blood levels, which are measured as a test for prostate cancer (see page 30). A recent study showed that the larger blood volume of obese men dilutes their PSA, making their PSA levels seem much lower than they really are. In other words, an obese patient could have prostate cancer, but his falsely low PSA readings would prevent him from being diagnosed at an early stage when the cancer was most curable. This means that obese patients are at a higher risk for developing more advanced prostate cancer because their true PSA levels are harder to detect. More research is needed on how PSA monitoring needs to be adjusted according to body weight.

Exercise

Studies have shown that by increasing exercise, you may be able to decrease cancer risk by up to 50 percent. See Chapter 14 for more information on how you can make exercise a part of your daily routine.

Stress Management

High stress levels can weaken your immune system and are associated with increased cancer risk. By reducing stress, you can reduce your risk of cancer and overall, live a healthier lifestyle. See Chapter 12 for techniques on stress management.

Prescription Medication to Prevent Prostate Cancer

In 1994, researchers in the US conducted a study to determine whether a drug called finasteride, which helps men with enlarged prostates urinate more easily, could prevent the development of prostate cancer. The reason investigators thought that finasteride might protect against prostate cancer is that it stops testosterone from being converted to dihydrotestosterone, the hormone responsible for allowing the prostate to grow and mature. It does this by inhibiting an enzyme called 5-alpha-reductase. Also, men who are missing 5-alpha-reductase due to a rare genetic disorder never seem to develop prostate cancer.

All of this evidence led US researchers to test whether finasteride could actually prevent the development of prostate cancer. They studied over 18,000 men, half of whom were given finasteride and half of whom were given a placebo (sugar pill) for 7 years. At the end of 7 years, all of the men underwent a prostate biopsy to determine whether or not they had prostate cancer. Researchers found that the rate of prostate cancer was significantly lower among the men who took finasteride (18 percent) compared to those who took a placebo (24 percent). This important study was published in 2003 in the prestigious medical journal the *New England Journal of Medicine*.

So why isn't every man taking finasteride as a preventive measure against prostate cancer? The reason is that a greater proportion of men who took finasteride in the study developed more aggressive forms of prostate cancer than the men taking the placebo. So it appears that, although finasteride may prevent you from getting prostate cancer in the first place, if you do get prostate cancer while on the drug you are likely to have a more aggressive tumour than if you hadn't taken it.

Since the 2003 study, many other studies have been published in an attempt to explain this phenomenon. Some research has suggested that this finding is false — that men who get prostate cancer while on finasteride do not develop a more aggressive tumour.

The US Food and Drug Administration (FDA) did their own investigation to see if finasteride and a newer but similar drug, dutasteride (Avodart), could in fact cause more aggressive forms of prostate cancer. After reviewing all of the data, the FDA concluded that indeed finasteride and dutasteride could cause patients to develop aggressive forms of prostate cancer if used for prevention. The FDA subsequently issued a safety warning about this potential effect of these drugs.

Therefore, it is not recommended to use finasteride or dutasteride for prostate cancer prevention purposes.

What Happens Next?

If you are reading this book because you want to learn more about how to prevent prostate cancer — good for you! The future does lie, to some extent, in your hands. Making some simple changes now, perhaps by losing weight or eating some unfamiliar but prostate-healthy foods, could be all it takes to prevent a life experience that most men could happily do without. Always check with your doctor when adding supplements and antioxidants to your diet. Although we have mentioned the benefits of various substances, there are times when they shouldn't be taken.

Chapter 3

tests and measurements

What Happens in This Chapter
- Prostate cancer screening
- Interpreting your PSA
- Tests for prostate cancer
- Understanding tumours

Several tests are available for finding out what is causing your urinary symptoms or your abnormal prostate cancer screening results. It's an anxious but constructive time because you're taking the first step toward getting some answers and ultimately feeling better.

Is It Cancer or Just Benign Enlargement?

If you have urinary symptoms you may be worrying that you have prostate cancer and delay going to see your doctor, afraid of what you might find. However, prostate cancer only rarely causes urinary symptoms, so it's much more likely that you are suffering from benign prostate enlargement, known medically as benign prostatic hyperplasia (BPH) (see Chapter 4).

! **[KEY POINT]**

Although benign prostate enlargement, or BPH, is not as serious as prostate cancer, you still can't afford to treat it lightly. Even though it's **benign** (meaning non-cancerous) you could develop more serious problems with your kidneys or bladder down the road, so be sure to see your doctor at the first sign of urinary symptoms.

On the other hand, many men who don't have urinary symptoms think they are "in the clear" and don't understand why they need to get screened regularly for prostate cancer. In fact, regular screening is very important *precisely because* early prostate cancer has virtually no symptoms and your cancer may not be discovered until it is far advanced.

Prostate Cancer Screening

The purpose of cancer screening is to detect cancer at an early stage, before any symptoms or signs are felt or seen. This is important because in many cancers, including prostate cancer, signs and symptoms tend to appear only once the cancer has grown to a large size or spread to other parts of the body (**metastasis**). This makes the cancer much more difficult to treat, so it's important to have tests that can catch it at an early stage and increase your chances of having your cancer treated successfully.

Prostate cancer screening consists of a blood test called prostate specific antigen (PSA) and a **digital rectal exam** (**DRE**), which is a physical examination of your prostate gland by your physician. Both these tests are described below.

If you are at higher risk of having prostate cancer—for example, if you have a family history of prostate cancer or you are African Canadian—it is advisable that you start having regular prostate cancer screening between the ages of 40 and 45. However, the exact age at which you should start having regular tests depends on how many of your family members are affected with prostate cancer, and you should discuss this with your physician.

Tests for Prostate Cancer

Digital Rectal Exam (DRE)
Touch tells a lot, which is why a digital rectal exam as part of an annual physical examination is recommended for all men over age 50.

For this test, the physician inserts a gloved, lubricated finger into the patient's **rectum** and feels the prostate for size, tenderness and nodules. When a prostate is enlarged, it often loses the central groove that separates its left and right lobes. Occasionally, the physician may feel a tumour on the prostate's surface as a hard, distinct lump.

Although DREs are useful, touch has its limits. With the widespread use of PSA testing, most prostate cancer is now detected in the early stages, before it can be felt on a DRE. It is also possible to have urinary tract symptoms due to enlargement of the part of the prostate that surrounds the urethra, even if it does not feel very enlarged on a DRE. The true value of a DRE comes from annual repetition as part of a general physical exam, so that your doctor has a baseline—a sense of what's normal for your body—from which to gauge possible changes.

PSA Test

Until the late 1980s, a digital rectal exam was the only way to detect prostate disease early. Now, annual screening and diagnostic procedures rely more on the PSA blood test. PSA is a protein produced by the prostate that helps keep semen in liquid form. Prostate cancer cells typically release more PSA into the bloodstream than healthy cells, so this test has been used for many years as an early warning of prostate cancer.

The amount of PSA is measured in nanograms (ng)—an unimaginably tiny *billionth* of a gram!—per millilitre (mL) of blood. In the past, a level of 4 ng/mL was generally considered normal, while a reading over 4 ng/mL was considered abnormal. However, we now know that interpreting PSA values isn't that simple, because some men with "abnormal" PSA may not have cancer, and—more importantly— some men with "normal" PSA may, in fact, have cancer. The accuracy of the PSA test is discussed in more detail below.

If your doctor has any concerns about the results of your PSA test, he or she will probably repeat it, and a prostate **biopsy** may be your next step (page 36).

How Accurate Is the PSA Test?

The Limitations of the PSA Test

A PSA test is a useful alert for prostate cancer, but, like all tests, it has limitations. The first downside is that it can give a **false positive**; in other words, it might suggest that you have cancer when in fact you don't. The reason for this is that other factors can increase the level of PSA in your blood. For example, if the prostate becomes inflamed (a condition called prostatitis), more PSA leaks into the bloodstream through the damaged lining of the gland, resulting in quite high PSA levels. Recent ejaculation or a biopsy, and some medications, can also artificially raise PSA levels.

Perhaps most significantly, PSA levels can also rise with benign prostate enlargement, or BPH, which occurs naturally in most men as they age, since there are more cells producing PSA. This realization has now led Dr Thomas Stamey, the Stanford urologist who laid the groundwork for the PSA test in the 1980s, to express doubts about the usefulness of the PSA test for detecting prostate cancer. He claims that rising PSA levels as men age are more likely to be caused by benign enlargement of the prostate than prostate cancer. This claim is highly controversial and is still being debated in the medical community.

On the flip side, the PSA test can also give a **false negative**; in other words, a man might still have prostate cancer even though his PSA is "normal." This was demonstrated quite dramatically in a recent, large study from the US. In the study, researchers tested the accuracy of the PSA test by asking healthy older men with "normal" PSA values (i.e., under 4.0 ng/mL) to have a prostate biopsy. They found that *the odds of having prostate cancer with a "normal" PSA value were as high as 1 in 4* (see table below).

PSA level (ng/mL)	Odds of having prostate cancer (confirmed by a biopsy)
undetectable to 0.5	1 in 15
0.6 to 1.0	1 in 10
1.1 to 2.0	1 in 6
2.1 to 3.0	1 in 4
3.1 to 4.0	1 in 6

Reference: Ian Thompson et al. New England Journal of Medicine, May 24, 2004.

Does the PSA Test Save Lives?

So, is prostate cancer screening with PSA worth the effort? Although detecting prostate cancer at an earlier stage seems to make sense, it may not be that simple.

Recently, two large clinical studies were done to see if prostate cancer screening actually saves lives or not—one in the US and the other in Europe. The US study involved over 75,000 men, some of whom underwent PSA screening and others who did not. After about 7 years, there was no difference in survival between the men who were screened and those who weren't. In contrast, the European study, which included over 160,000 men, found a better rate of survival among prostate cancer patients if they had undergone PSA screening.

Why the difference in the two studies? The main reason was that the men in the US study who were assigned to the "no screening" group didn't listen and went ahead with a PSA test anyway. This caused what was referred to as "contamination" of the data, making it impossible to compare men who'd had a PSA test with those who had not. In effect, the study was comparing groups of men who had all had the test! On the other hand, although the European study did not have this problem, the advantage of the PSA test was small. But, after several more years of following these men, the European study found that PSA screening had a greater life-saving advantage.

To sort out the confusion, the US Preventive Services Task Force (USPSTF) in healthcare was put in charge of reviewing all the science to try and make a final ruling on the benefits (or not) of PSA testing. The USPSTF concluded that PSA screening did not improve the chances of surviving prostate cancer. However, this did not end the debate. Many experts criticized the USPSTF's methodology for reviewing the studies. They had overlooked the "contamination" in the US study and, said experts, dismissed other studies showing a benefit of PSA screening, for "technical reasons."

In response, the American Society of Clinical Oncology—the largest association for cancer specialists in North America—set out to review the evidence in a more balanced way. Dr Nam was asked to form a committee and co-chair the review. This group of doctors concluded that there was good scientific evidence to consider PSA screening for men who are healthy and young. The results of this review are published in the *Journal of Clinical Oncology*. PSA screening will remain a controversial subject and, despite millions of dollars invested in clinical trials, we still do not have a definitive answer on whether it saves lives or not. This has to be balanced against the fact that the earlier prostate cancer is detected, the better the chances are for a cure.

So what's the bottom line on PSA? Most physicians agree that although the PSA test is not as accurate as we had once hoped, it's still the only test out there that *can* detect prostate cancer early, and that makes it the best thing we've got so far.

Making PSA Tests Better

In the meantime, scientists continue working to make PSA tests more accurate. For example, one approach focuses on the amount of **free PSA**—PSA not bound to protein—in the blood. Free-PSA testing appears to be significantly more accurate at detecting cancer in some patients with particular PSA values, such as the 4 to 10 ng/mL range, and can eliminate the need for some prostate biopsies.

The rate of change of PSA over time (called **PSA velocity**, or **PSAV**) can also be a more accurate indication of whether you have cancer. One important study

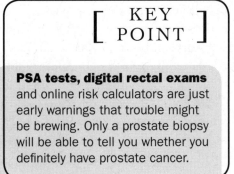

[**KEY POINT**]

PSA tests, digital rectal exams and online risk calculators are just early warnings that trouble might be brewing. Only a prostate biopsy will be able to tell you whether you definitely have prostate cancer.

found that if your PSA levels increase by 0.75 ng/mL or more per year, your chances of having prostate cancer are high.

Another interesting approach is the so-called **prostate cancer risk calculators**. These are discussed in the next section.

Prostate Cancer Risk Calculators

Prostate cancer researchers have developed computer programs that work with the existing PSA test, but boost its accuracy by adding a few more factors into the equation. As discussed in Chapter 1, age, ethnicity and a family history of prostate cancer all increase a man's risk of having prostate cancer. Prostate cancer risk calculators crunch all the numbers—including the results of the DRE exam and PSA tests—and give each man his individual risk of having prostate cancer.

Compared with using PSA and DRE results alone, these calculators are much more reliable for predicting prostate cancer because they also take into account your age, race, family history of cancer and other factors that could affect your cancer risk.

If you are interested in trying these calculators for yourself, here are a couple of examples:

National Cancer Institute Prostate Cancer Risk Calculator (US)
This online tool uses age, ethnicity, PSA level, family history of prostate cancer, the DRE result and previous biopsy results to estimate the risk of prostate cancer: http://www.compass.fhcrc.org/edrnnci/bin/calculator/main.asp?t=prostate&sub=disclaimer&v=prostate&m=&x=Prostate%20Cancer

Sunnybrook Prostate Cancer Risk Calculator (Canada)
This online tool, developed by Dr Nam and his research colleagues at the University of Toronto, takes into account symptoms and ratio of free to total PSA, in addition to age, ethnicity, PSA level, family history of prostate cancer and the DRE result to estimate the risk of prostate cancer: http://www.prostaterisk.ca

(see Figure 3–1). Dr Nam and his research team recently tested this calculator among different patients and found it to be highly accurate, and better than the US-based calculator.

Figure 3–1 Sunnybrook Prostate Risk Calculator

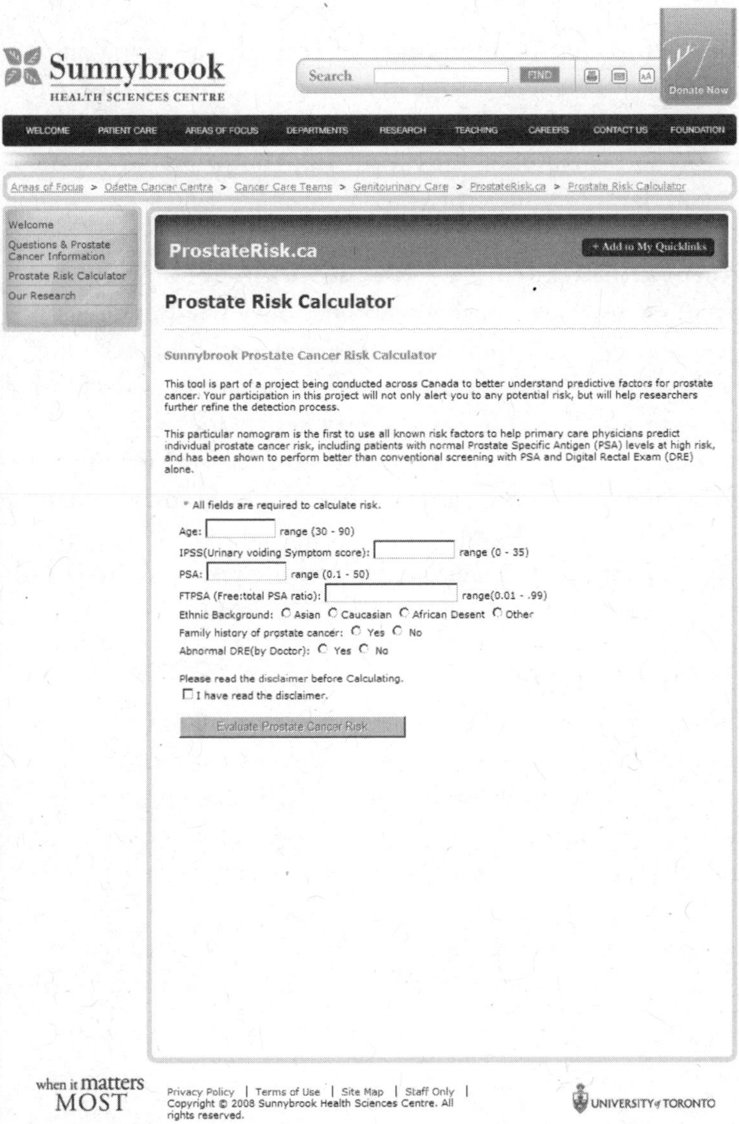

European Prostate Cancer Risk Calculator

This calculator is based on patients who participated in the European prostate cancer screening study and is similar to the US- and Canadian-based calculators (www.prostatecancer-riskcalculator.com).

It is important to bear in mind that such calculators give you your *risk* of having cancer—they give no guarantees, either way. If you do try one out, be sure to discuss your results with your doctor, and remember, only a prostate biopsy will tell you whether you definitely have prostate cancer.

Other Tumour Markers for Prostate Cancer

For the past 30 years, several researchers have tried to develop new screening tools for prostate cancer that could replace or enhance the PSA test. Recently, Canadian researchers developed a new urine test called PCA3 that could help achieve this goal. It is based on a prostate cancer gene called *PCA3*, which appears to be overactive in prostate cancer cells compared to cells that are normal. This overactivity can be measured in urine, using the PCA3 test. At this time, clinical use of the test is limited, and your doctor will order it only in certain circumstances.

Prostate Biopsy

The only way to determine whether you definitely have prostate cancer or not is to have a prostate biopsy. This procedure involves obtaining a small piece of prostate tissue with a needle. The tissue is then processed and examined by another doctor, called a **pathologist**, to identify any prostate cancer cells.

Ultrasound is used during the prostate biopsy to create an image of the prostate and help the physician guide the biopsy needle into the prostate gland. The ultrasound probe and biopsy device are inserted into your rectum, so the procedure is called **transrectal ultrasound (TRUS)**-guided biopsy. The ultrasound image will also allow your physician to assess the size of your prostate gland and see any obvious tumours, although in most cases the tumours are microscopic and cannot be seen. For this reason, your physician will take several biopsies randomly throughout the gland to increase the chances of detecting any cancer tissue.

With the ultrasound probe to guide his or her actions from a monitor, the physician uses the probe's spring-loaded hollow needles to quickly pierce the rectal wall, enter into the prostate and retrieve multiple cylinders of tissue 1.5 mm (1/32 inch) in diameter. The exact number of samples taken will depend on your own situation, but in general, expect about 8 to

! **[KEY POINT]**

About 7 to 10 days before your biopsy, you will need to stop taking ASA (e.g., Aspirin), other pain relief medications (such as ibuprofen) and vitamin E, because these may make you bleed more heavily afterward. If you are taking a blood-thinning medication (such as Coumadin, Fragmin or low-molecular-weight heparins), ask the doctor who prescribed it for instructions. Depending on the blood-thinning medication you're taking and your reasons for being on it, you may have to stop your drug or take another medication to reverse its effects.
You should also tell your physician if you have problems with your heart valves or have prosthetics that require **antibiotics** before any type of medical or dental procedure. In this case, you may need to take additional antibiotics before your biopsy.

12 passes. Don't worry—you will be given a **local anesthetic** to numb the area first. The samples are then sent to a pathology lab for analysis. The whole procedure takes about 15 to 20 minutes.

Preparing for a Biopsy

A TRUS-guided biopsy has a few more risks than other tests you'll undergo because it's more invasive. Rest assured that every precaution is taken to minimize your discomfort and risk of infection. The night before the biopsy, you may be asked to give yourself an enema or take a laxative to clean out your lower bowel. This will help make the biopsy site clean. In addition, you'll be prescribed an antibiotic that should be taken before and after the biopsy until the course of medication is complete.

After the Biopsy

After the procedure, you may experience bleeding from your rectum or penis, and there may be blood in your stool, urine or semen. This can last for up to 2 weeks or more. Don't be alarmed by this; it is quite normal.

Some men feel a little discomfort in the prostate following the procedure when the local anesthetic wears off, so you may want to have the option of taking the day off work. However, most men are able to leave the hospital on their own without any difficulty and return to work right away. Pain relief such as acetaminophen (e.g., Tylenol) will quickly relieve some of the bruised, achy feeling.

Repeat Biopsies

Sometimes, a repeat biopsy is recommended, even if the first results are negative for cancer. There are several reasons your physician might want you to undergo additional biopsies.

Because only a small percentage of the total prostate gland is sampled, the first biopsy could miss the prostate cancer in the gland. Indeed, it has been found that 15 to 30 percent of prostate cancers can be detected from a repeat biopsy after the first biopsy came out negative.

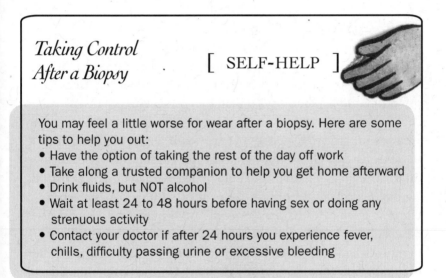

Taking Control After a Biopsy   [SELF-HELP]

You may feel a little worse for wear after a biopsy. Here are some tips to help you out:
- Have the option of taking the rest of the day off work
- Take along a trusted companion to help you get home afterward
- Drink fluids, but NOT alcohol
- Wait at least 24 to 48 hours before having sex or doing any strenuous activity
- Contact your doctor if after 24 hours you experience fever, chills, difficulty passing urine or excessive bleeding

Another reason for doing a second biopsy is that non-cancerous but abnormal cells might be found in the first biopsy. Men with this non-cancerous condition, known as **atypical small acinar cell proliferation (ASAP)**, have up to a 1 in 2 risk of having or developing prostate cancer, so a repeat biopsy is essential. **Prostatic intraepithelial neoplasia (PIN)** was once thought to be a precursor to prostate cancer and, therefore, required close attention and repeat biopsies. However, PIN is now known not to be a precursor, making a repeat biopsy unnecessary.

Some specialists favour a procedure called **saturation biopsy**, in which you go to sleep under a **general anesthetic** and a larger number of samples are taken. This can be helpful in finding prostate cancer in cases where multiple biopsies have shown no evidence of cancer. You and your **urologist** will need to decide if this option is right for you.

Complications From Biopsies
Although a prostate biopsy is considered a safe and well-tolerated procedure, a small proportion of men do develop complications. The most common ones are bleeding, urinary infection and an inability to urinate (retention).

In a recent study, Dr Nam and his team were the first group to demonstrate that complication rates are on the rise. Based on the entire population of Ontario men who'd had a prostate biopsy over a 10-year period, the study found that serious complication rates had risen from 1 to 4 percent. Other studies have subsequently confirmed Dr Nam's results by studying men undergoing prostate biopsies in the US and Europe. These results should not discourage patients from having a prostate biopsy, since it is a very safe procedure. If you do undergo a prostate biopsy, keep in mind that complications may occur and, if you have any of the symptoms listed above, speak to your doctor immediately so that he or she can treat you promptly.

Understanding Tumours

Your biopsy results may take anywhere from 3 to 14 days, depending on the hospital. A pathologist will examine your tissue samples and let your physician know whether or not you have cancer. If the pathologist finds evidence of cancer, he or she can also tell your physician how aggressive the cancer appears to be.

Your Gleason Score

If you have prostate cancer, your Gleason score—based on the appearance of your cancer cells under a microscope—will help your physicians decide how aggressive your cancer is and what treatment you need.

Gleason score	Percentage of men with prostate cancer	What this means
5	<1%	Very non-aggressive No treatment is necessary
6	40%	Considered non-aggressive Cancer cells may spread Can do nothing, or treat with surgery or radiation
7	45%	Moderately aggressive Needs to be treated to prevent spread Surgery or radiation effective
8 to 10	15%	Very aggressive Needs prompt treatment May need to treat with multiple treatments: surgery, radiation and medication

How Aggressive Is Your Cancer?

In simple terms, an "aggressive" cancer is one that is likely to spread rapidly to other parts of your body and threaten your life. To decide how aggressive a case of prostate cancer is, physicians use a grading system called the **Gleason score**. The pathologist who examines your tumour cells will assign the Gleason score—usually a number between 2 and 10. Patients with a Gleason score of 10 have a very aggressive-appearing prostate cancer, while in patients with a

Gleason score of 2 to 5 the cancer appears very benign. The higher the score, the greater the chance that the cancer has already spread (see More Detail box on the previous page) or will come back after surgery or radiation.

The other two factors that your physician considers are your PSA level and the specific stage of the cancer (how large it is and whether it has spread outside the prostate gland—see the More Detail box on the next page.). As is the case with the Gleason score, patients with a higher PSA level have more aggressive cancer. Patients with a PSA of 20 ng/mL or more have a poorer prognosis than patients with levels below 20 ng/mL. Patients with a higher stage of cancer also have a poorer prognosis. The combination of the Gleason score, PSA level and stage are used to assess the overall risk of the prostate cancer spreading and metastasizing, and can be summarized as (1) low risk, (2) intermediate risk, and (3) high risk.

Has Your Cancer Spread?

Your treatment will also depend on the **stage** of your prostate cancer, that is, whether it has already spread outside your prostate gland. Prostate cancer can spread to areas immediately beside the gland, to lymph nodes, to your bones or to other organs.

The most common way that physicians stage prostate cancer is the TNM staging system (see More Detail box opposite). TNM stands for the three stages that cancer moves through as it spreads: "T" for tumour, "N" for (lymph) nodes, and "M" for **metastases** (cancer growths in bones and other organs).

The "T" is usually assessed by a digital rectal exam by your physician. The "N" and "M" components need to be assessed by X-ray tests such as a **CAT scan** (page 44). You may not need these additional tests if your cancer has a low risk of spreading—that is, if you have both a low Gleason score and a low PSA level. The decision on whether further staging tests are needed will be made by your **oncologist**, based on how your tumour looks.

TNM Staging System (2002) [MORE DETAIL]

This system helps describe the stage of development of your cancer.

Stage   Description

Stage	Description
T1	The tumour cannot be felt or seen using ultrasound.
T1a	Cancer cells are "accidentally" found in 5 percent or less of tissue samples from prostate surgery for benign disease.
T1b	Cancer cells are found in more than 5 percent of sample tissue from surgery.
T1c	Cancer cells are identified by needle biopsy performed because of high PSA.
T2	The cancer is confined to the prostate but can be felt as a small, well-defined nodule.
T2a	Tumours are in half a prostate lobe.
T2b	Tumours are in more than half a prostate lobe.
T2c	Tumours are in both lobes.
T3	Tumour extends through the prostate capsule.
T3a	Tumour extends through the capsule on one side only.
T3b	Tumour extends through the capsule on two sides.
T3c	Tumour extends into the seminal vesicles.
T4	Tumour is fixed to or invades adjacent structures (other than the seminal vesicles).
T4a	Tumour has spread to the neck of the bladder, the external sphincter or the rectum.
T4b	Tumour has spread to the floor and/or the wall of the pelvis.
N0	Regional lymph nodes are still cancer-free.
N1	A small tumour is in a single pelvic lymph node.
N2	A medium-sized tumour is in one lymph node, or small tumours are in several nodes.
N3	A large tumour is in one or more lymph nodes.
M0	Cancer has not spread beyond regional lymph nodes.
M1a	Cancer has spread to lymph nodes distant from regional nodes.
M1b	Cancer has invaded the bones.
M1c	Cancer has spread to other sites.

If your cancer is still confined to the prostate gland, you may be eligible for **radical prostatectomy** (removal of your prostate gland). Your urologist will discuss this with you.

If your cancer has spread beyond the prostate gland, or metastasized, then radical prostatectomy will not be a useful treatment strategy. Other treatments, such as radiation and hormonal medications, are available in this case, and do provide good cancer control.

Finding Tumours Outside the Prostate

If your physician is concerned that the cancer may have spread locally, he or she can send you for a number of high-tech tests to confirm this. Usually, the results take between 1 and 3 weeks, and if they show that the cancer has spread, your physician will be able to adjust your treatment accordingly (see Chapter 5).

Computerized Axial Tomography (CAT) Scans

Typically, CAT scans are used to try to detect whether cancer has spread from the prostate to nearby clusters of lymph nodes. Instead of a tube being placed in you, this time it's the other way around. During this test, you lie on your back inside a long rotating tube that takes narrow-beam, 360-degree, thinly layered X-ray pictures of your body. A high-speed computer stacks each image slice one on top of the other, like a deck of cards, and produces a 3-dimensional image of your abdomen.

Before the CAT scan, you may receive an injection of special dye to heighten the contrast and thus improve the image quality of your veins, arteries, kidneys, liver and spleen. The injection may cause a feeling of spreading warmth and, possibly, itching as it circulates throughout your body. If you have allergies, inform the radiotherapist before the procedure, since it may be safer to avoid the dye. After the test, increase your intake of fluids to flush out your system. Water and juice are good choices.

Magnetic Resonance Imaging (MRI)

This device measures the amount of magnetic energy given off by various cells. The MRI combines an extremely powerful magnet with radio waves to create high-quality images. People who have metallic implants, such as joint replacement implants, orthopedic rods and nails for fracture repair, or a pacemaker, cannot undergo this test. Also, people who can't tolerate lying motionless in an enclosed tube for the length of the procedure, which may take from 20 minutes to an hour, will not be able to have an MRI. All patients fill out an in-depth questionnaire before their MRI to bring these issues to light.

Bone Scan

The purpose of this scan is to see whether your prostate cancer has spread to your bones. A small amount of **radioisotope** is injected into your bloodstream while you're lying on your back. The radioactive solution is attracted to areas of your skeleton where changes have taken place, for example, due to fractures, infections or arthritis, or other bone diseases. A device is then passed over your body to measure the tiny amount of radioactivity the isotopes emit. If the cancer has spread to nearby bone, then it will appear as a "hot spot," since the isotope concentrates in these areas. The test has no unwanted aftereffects; the amount of radioactivity involved is safe and doesn't raise your risk of developing other types of cancer.

What Happens Next?

Now that you and your physician have a clearer understanding of your condition, you can work together to take control of your health. You must decide what course of treatment is best for you, and Chapter 5 can help you make up your mind.

Chapter 4

benign prostatic hyperplasia

What Happens in This Chapter
- BPH causes and symptoms
- Treatment options, including watchful waiting, drugs and surgery
- Reasons for recommending TURP
- Step-by-step guide to TURP
- What to expect afterward
- Measuring success

Urinary symptoms in men over 50 are usually caused by benign enlargement of the prostate gland—a condition known as benign prostatic hyperplasia, or BPH. This benign enlargement of the prostate is a normal part of aging for many men and is a completely different condition than prostate cancer. You can choose to treat BPH with drugs or surgery, a procedure known as transurethral resection of the prostate (TURP), or simply nothing at all—a "wait and see" approach.

Why a Chapter on Benign Prostate Enlargement?

As described in Chapter 1, the three most common conditions that can affect your prostate are the following: infection of the prostate, or prostatitis; prostate cancer, which is covered in the rest of this book; and benign prostate enlargement, or benign prostatic hyperplasia (BPH), which is discussed in this chapter. When you buy this book you may be having urinary symptoms and still be uncertain what is wrong with your prostate. In case it turns out that you only have BPH, not cancer, this chapter is for you.

Basics of Benign Prostate Enlargement

At around age 50, the prostate begins to enlarge as a result of a condition called benign prostatic hyperplasia. This happens when benign clusters of cells called **adenomas** begin to form within the central zone of the prostate (see Figure 4–1). Over time, these multiply (hyperplasia) and thus slowly increase the size of the prostate. As it enlarges, the prostate slowly compresses the urethra, and urination may become difficult.

Whatever the causes of prostate enlargement (see More Detail box on page 51), the condition can make passing urine (**voiding**) difficult. These symptoms are known collectively as **lower urinary tract symptoms** (**LUTS**).

If you are having trouble voiding, it is likely because your urethra and **bladder neck** are being squeezed, or constricted. In BPH, this constriction happens very gradually, so you might not realize it at first. See if this scenario sounds familiar:

Figure 4–1A. A Normal Prostate Gland

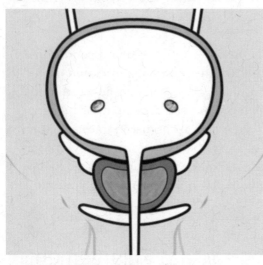

The prostate gland sits beneath the bladder. It consists of an inner zone and an outer zone, and is divided into left and right lobes.

Figure 4–1B. Benign Prostatic Hyperplasia (BPH)

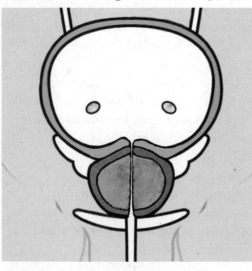

BPH occurs when the cells in the inner zone of the prostate start to multiply and grow. The growing prostate may compress the urethra and the bladder, making urination difficult.

One day, you notice that your urine stream isn't as forceful as it used to be. Eventually, there's a delay in starting the urine flow, and no matter how hard you try, the flow tapers off to a dribbling conclusion. Or perhaps you experience the phenomenon captured by the apt French phrase *pis en deux*, which describes passing a second large volume of urine after the first flow stops.

More annoying still are the storage symptoms that develop as a result of the hard work your bladder has to do to overcome the voiding problems. The strain of not being able to fully empty your bladder makes you go to the bathroom urgently and more frequently. After you relieve yourself, your bladder still feels partly full. The bladder's signals to urinate are so strong that you are repeatedly woken up during the night, a condition called **nocturia**. Recognize the pattern? For most men, this is an all-too-familiar description of how BPH encroaches on their quality of life.

[! KEY POINT]

The symptoms of prostate enlargement are lower urinary tract symptoms (LUTS). They include:
- A sudden, urgent need to urinate (**urgency**)
- A weak or intermittent urinary stream
- Not being able to urinate at all (**urinary retention**)
- Straining when urinating
- Hesitation before urine flow starts
- Feeling the bladder hasn't emptied completely
- Dribbling or leakage
- Painful urination

You may also occasionally experience:
- Blood in the urine (**hematuria**) or a urinary tract infection

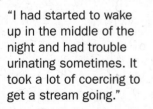

"I had started to wake up in the middle of the night and had trouble urinating sometimes. It took a lot of coercing to get a stream going."

RAY

BPH can cause other problems too. Urine that has been sitting in the bladder for a long time may form crystals that grow into stones. Passing a stone through the urethra is an experience few men forget and could lead to the need for surgery. This "old" urine can also become a breeding ground for common bacteria and cause infections of the bladder and urinary tract. One sign of an infection is a burning sensation when urinating. If you've been diagnosed with BPH and have been experiencing repeated bladder and urinary tract infections, surgery may be a better option than recurring bouts of illness and prescriptions for antibiotics.

Another symptom of BPH is acute urinary retention, with which you suddenly lose the ability to urinate. The bladder fills up and becomes extremely painful. The trigger for acute urinary retention can be as simple as constipation, prolonged bed rest or standing in the cold with an overly full bladder. A minor infection may also cause the urethra to swell or the prostate to enlarge just enough to complete the blockage. The most effective immediate treatment for this urgent complication is for a doctor to insert a **catheter** (a thin, hollow tube) into the bladder to drain the urine (see page 139).

Occasionally, as a result of weak signals between the spinal cord and bladder, urine retention can become chronic. A man's bladder can fill up painlessly over a period of months (even years!) until it expands to many times its normal size. He may experience vague abdominal and pelvic discomfort and only pass urine in small quantities. Every once in a while, there may be leakage, but generally the man is unaware that his bladder is overly full. Very rarely, the pressure from the bladder can rise to such an extent that urine is forced back along the ureters to the kidneys, causing harm. Once again, catheterization is the immediate first step to recovery, usually followed by surgery. However, a severely enlarged or distended bladder may never return to its normal size and may have trouble contracting and emptying properly in the future.

New Theories for an Old Problem [MORE DETAIL]

There are a number of theories about why prostate enlargement happens. The most popular theory blames the principal male **hormone**, **testosterone**. After puberty and well into old age, the prostate is routinely bathed with testosterone. Once inside the prostate, testosterone is converted into an even more powerful hormone, **dihydrotestosterone** (**DHT**), which stimulates the prostate's glandular cells to grow during puberty. Not surprisingly, DHT is the chief suspect in mid- and late-life prostatic glandular enlargement.

However, some experts place the blame on DHT's female counterpart, **estrogen**, which is normally present at low levels in men. The relative proportion of estrogen increases as men age and produce less testosterone. This change in hormonal proportions could possibly trigger prostate enlargement.

The "late bloomers" theory argues that certain types of prostate cells only become active later in life, when they become sensitive to DHT and other growth signals. Another theory claims that some of the glandular cells might not know when to call it quits, disobeying normal self-destruct orders and multiplying instead.

Whatever the exact mechanism, genetics may help to explain why some men develop BPH and others don't. Studies have shown that men who need surgery for enlarged prostates often have a family history—that is, they have a father or brother with the same problem. However, a "BPH gene" has not yet been identified.

Tests and Measurements for BPH

There is a specific group of tests that your doctor will want you to undergo if you start experiencing lower urinary tract symptoms. While some of them may be uncomfortable, they can tell your physician a lot about what the problem is and how best to help you.

AUA Symptom Score

Along with a physical examination, your answers to this questionnaire designed by the American Urological Association will help your physician gain a more accurate understanding of the nature and severity of your urinary symptoms. The **AUA symptom score** is particularly helpful in diagnosing BPH and deciding whether treatment is a good idea. It is also helpful in monitoring how well you respond to treatment.

Uroflow

During your assessment, the doctor may send you for a **uroflow test**. The test measures how fast and how well you can empty your bladder.

Abdominal Ultrasound

This imaging tool is used to see inside the kidneys and bladder. **Ultrasound** works on the same principle as marine SONAR: sound waves are emitted and allowed to bounce off objects in their path. The echoes created from the bounced waves produce an image of what the ultrasound signal bumped into. The ultrasound probe works at very high frequencies (well beyond human hearing) to provide fine detail at a range of several centimetres. The image that the ultrasound test produces can reveal stones and other problems with the kidneys, ureters or bladder. This test is often used to rule out other possible reasons for urinary tract symptoms. It has no side effects and is non-invasive, which means that no equipment will penetrate your outer layer of skin.

Cystoscopy

A **cystoscope** is a slender, flexible, fibre-optic device that is passed down your urethra, through the prostate and into your bladder. It allows your urologist to look directly at your urinary tract. The reason for doing **cystoscopy** is to rule out other causes for your symptoms. Cystoscopy can identify abnormalities in your bladder and prostate gland that other tests may not be able to reveal, such as **urethral stricture** (narrowing of the urethra) or **bladder stones**, which can mimic the symptoms of prostate enlargement. It also helps your urologist map out your specific anatomy for any future surgical treatments that may be required.

Your urethra will be numbed with an anesthetic gel before the cystoscope is inserted. For the first 24 hours after cystoscopy you may experience minor irritation or bleeding when you urinate.

Treatment Options for BPH

If you have BPH, there are three treatment options to consider: watchful waiting, medication and surgery. The pros and cons of these options are summarized in the chart on page 63. Most commonly, physicians tend to start with the least invasive options. Surgery is usually reserved for men whose symptoms do not improve with medication, or when BPH starts to cause serious medical problems.

Watchful Waiting
Watchful waiting is the medical term for a "wait-and-see" approach. You and your physician will keep a close eye on your symptoms but do nothing unless something changes.

Scientific studies involving large numbers of men suggest that BPH symptoms improve or disappear on their own in 20 to 50 percent of cases. Therefore, many men do not need any treatment. However, about a third of those who choose to wait and see will experience progressive worsening of their symptoms, and some may eventually lose the ability to empty their bladder. The 10-year risk for developing acute urinary retention (see page 50) is about 13 percent—or odds of slightly better than 1 in 10. The risk for requiring surgery for BPH is about 5 percent (or odds of 1 in 20). These low probabilities make watchful waiting quite attractive, especially when BPH symptoms are mild and not too bothersome.

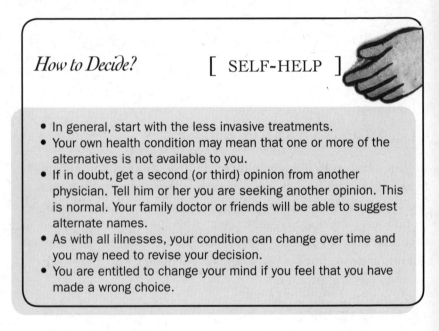

How to Decide?　　　[SELF-HELP]

- In general, start with the less invasive treatments.
- Your own health condition may mean that one or more of the alternatives is not available to you.
- If in doubt, get a second (or third) opinion from another physician. Tell him or her you are seeking another opinion. This is normal. Your family doctor or friends will be able to suggest alternate names.
- As with all illnesses, your condition can change over time and you may need to revise your decision.
- You are entitled to change your mind if you feel that you have made a wrong choice.

Living With Untreated Prostate Enlargement
Most men adjust to mild urinary symptoms—a visit to the washroom before leaving home, scouting out the public lavatory at the mall, taking the aisle seat at the movies, and reducing fluid intake after dinner or before bedtime.

Certain medications can aggravate BPH symptoms. If you have allergies or catch a cold, you'll have to think twice about taking non-prescription medications known as **adrenergics**, because they mimic the effects of **adrenaline** (also called **epinephrine**). This is the "fight-or-flight" hormone that evolved in mammals to speed up the body for coping with emergencies such as outrunning a lion or avoiding an oncoming car. Many decongestants contain a synthetic version of adrenaline, called **pseudoephedrine**, which relaxes the lung's bronchial passages, stimulates the heart rate and constricts blood vessels. Another problem with adrenergics is that they constrict muscles in the prostate and bladder, making it harder to urinate. **Antihistamines**, such as **diphenhydramine** (Benadryl), can also slow urine flow in some men.

Anyone who has BPH and **hypertension** (high blood pressure) or **congestive heart disease** and is taking **diuretics**, such as chlorthalidone or hydrochlorothiazide, should discuss the risks and benefits of this drug regimen with his doctor. Diuretics (also called "water pills") decrease the amount of fluid in your body by encouraging the kidneys to produce large quantities of urine. This might be a good thing for hypertension, but clearly there's a conflict for someone who has lower urinary tract symptoms or is prone to urinary retention. However, no one should stop taking diuretics without medical supervision since these drugs are an important treatment for cardiovascular disease.

Drug Therapy

Medication has become a popular treatment choice for BPH. In the United States, the number of prescriptions written monthly for BPH drugs increased from less than 400,000 to more than one million between 1993 and 1996. The obvious advantage of drug therapy is that it provides effective relief of BPH symptoms without surgery.

The prostate is made up of muscle fibres and glandular cells. Both types of tissue enlarge and multiply as the prostate grows, so medications for prostate symptoms fall into two groups: drugs that relax the prostate's muscle tissue (**alpha-blockers**) and drugs that shrink the glandular tissue (**5-alpha-reductase inhibitors**).

Alpha-blockers

As we discussed earlier in this chapter, as the prostate enlarges, the muscular fibres in the gland become larger and squeeze the urethra more tightly (see Figure 4–1B). Alpha-blockers relax these muscle fibres, allowing urine to flow along the urethra more easily. Studies show that they improve both the symptoms of prostate disease and the actual measurable urine flow. The advantage of alpha-blockers is that they work fast. The downside of alpha-blockers is that they started out as blood-pressure-lowering drugs and can cause symptoms such as faintness and dizziness. However, a newer generation of alpha-blockers such as tamsulosin (Flomax) and alfuzosin (Xatral) appear to target the prostate more than the blood vessels and thus are just as effective but cause less dizziness. Alfuzosin appears to have a better side-effect profile than tamsulosin.

A word of caution about tamsulosin, and possibly all alpha-blockers. Tamsulosin may cause serious problems for men who have cataract surgery. Recent studies have shown that tamsulosin is associated with a condition called **floppy iris syndrome** that arises after cataract surgery and that could lead to bleeding and blindness. For this reason, tamsulosin needs to be stopped many months before surgery. The advice here is to tell your eye doctor about all drugs you are on before cataract surgery, especially alpha-blockers of any kind.

5-alpha-reductase Inhibitors

These medicines shrink the prostate by targeting its glandular tissue. They do this by blocking the production of the hormone dihydrotestosterone (DHT). This "high-octane" version of testosterone appears to encourage glandular cells in the prostate to grow and multiply. The 5-alpha-reductase inhibitors currently available are finasteride (Proscar) and dutasteride (Avodart), with several more in development. Although finasteride and dutasteride come with an FDA warning when used for prostate cancer prevention (see Chapter 2), these drugs are still appropriate for treatment of BPH.

Finasteride appears to be most helpful for men who have very large, mainly glandular prostates. In these men, finasteride can reduce prostate volume by up to 20 percent and reduce the need for surgery by half (from 8 to 4 percent). The downside of finasteride is that it can take up to 6 months to provide relief and does not appear to be as effective as the alpha-blockers in improving symptoms and urinary flow. Dutasteride is a more potent inhibitor of DHT and works more quickly, reducing DHT by about 90 percent within a few weeks. Because DHT has few functions outside the prostate, these drugs have few side effects. Sexual dysfunction (low sexual drive, **impotence** and decreased ejaculation) is the main one and affects about 3 percent of men, although this improves over the first year in about half of men treated.

Combination Therapy

If you're wondering why your doctor has put you on two different medicines for your BPH, it may be because he or she has been keeping up with the latest scientific studies.

When alpha-blockers and the 5-alpha-reductase inhibitor finasteride were first introduced, several studies compared how effective they were. These early studies found that alpha-blockers alone worked better than finasteride alone or a combination of alpha-blockers and finasteride. As a result, as one might expect, physicians prescribed a lot more alpha-blockers than finasteride. However, these studies used the drugs for only 1 year.

Recently, a long-term study was conducted where patients took the drugs for more than 4 years. This study was also more useful because it looked at whether these drugs could prevent the serious conditions that could happen as BPH gradually got worse, including more uncomfortable symptoms, kidney failure, urinary infections and bleeding. The scientists running this study found that a combination of an alpha-blocker (doxazosin) and finasteride was best at preventing the progression of BPH, compared with a sugar pill (placebo), doxazosin alone or finasteride alone. This has resulted in a dramatic increase in the use of finasteride along with an alpha-blocker for treating BPH.

Triple Combination Therapy

Recently a study has looked at whether adding a third drug, called an anticholinergic, to an alpha-blocker and a 5-alpha-reductase inhibitor could do a better job at controlling the uncomfortable symptoms of BPH. The anticholinergic drug tolterodine (Detrol) reduces the spasms of the bladder muscle wall, thereby lessening the frequent urge to empty the bladder experienced by men with BPH. The study found that BPH-related symptoms improved most when used in this triple combination approach. Although this is all good news, bear in mind that anticholinergics such as tolterodine can actually *cause* bladder problems and episodes of urinary retention, so it's important that you let your urologist's office know right away if your symptoms get worse after he or she prescribes tolterodine.

BPH Medications and Potential Side Effects

Drugs	Common side effects
Alpha-blockers	
e.g., alfuzosin (Xatral), doxazosin (Cardura), tamsulosin (Flomax), terazosin (Hytrin)	Dizziness or faintness after rising from a lying or sitting position, headaches, nausea, heart palpitations, stuffy nose, tiredness or weakness
	RARELY—heart failure and stroke
5-alpha-reductase inhibitors	
e.g., finasteride (Proscar), dutasteride (Avodart)	Erectile dysfunction, loss of libido, ejaculation disorder

The Downsides of Drug Therapy

So if these medications are effective, why does anyone opt for surgery? For one thing, although alpha-blockers and 5-alpha-reductase inhibitors can slow the progression of the disease, either alone or in combination, studies show that this does not work for all men. Symptoms can worsen during drug treatment; in particular, acute urinary retention can still occur, despite combination therapy. And symptoms return soon after you stop taking the drugs, so you may need to take medication for the rest of your life. Also, some of the drugs aren't currently covered by public or private drug plans, so this approach may prove to be expensive. Some men also find side effects, such as dizziness, ejaculatory problems or nasal congestion, troublesome. Although drug therapy alone can be an effective method of treating BPH, regular checkups with your doctor are a must if this is the route you choose.

! [KEY POINT]

A word of warning about finasteride, dutasteride and the PSA test. When you start taking these drugs, your PSA level should fall because, as your prostate shrinks, the cells that produce PSA also shrink. Within 6 months, your PSA level should fall by 50 percent or more. If your PSA does NOT drop by 50 percent within 6 months, this might indicate that you have prostate cancer since, in theory, prostate cancer cells do not shrink as much as normal prostate cells, keeping your PSA levels high. So what does this mean in practical terms? First, ensure your urologist measures your PSA level within 6 months of starting these drugs. Second, if your PSA level does not drop as expected, you may need to undergo a prostate biopsy to rule out the possibility of having prostate cancer.

> Although many food supplements and herbs claim to be good for prostate health, only one—**saw palmetto**—has even got close to being supported by science. This herb has been described as "the old man's friend" and has been used to treat BPH for centuries. A few small studies have shown that it seems to be as effective as (and work in a similar way to) the prescription drug finasteride. However, a more recent, well-designed study published in the prestigious *New England Journal of Medicine* found that saw palmetto was little better than the placebo. Vitamin E may also reduce the symptoms of BPH, although more studies need to be done to prove this.

Surgery

Surgery for BPH is called **TURP (transurethral resection of the prostate)**. It is considered elective—that is, it's your choice if and when you have the procedure. For many men, their choice depends on how well they can put up with reduced urinary flow and frequent urination (especially during the night). Some can tolerate urinary tract symptoms with little difficulty; others cannot. However, you may not really have a choice under certain circumstances, such as if you experience a decline in kidney function, repeated episodes of blood in your urine, multiple urinary tract infections and bladder stones. Surgery is also a good option if you develop **diverticula**, abnormal pockets of tissue in the bladder that can trap urine and cause infection.

What Happens During TURP

If you're undergoing TURP, you will need to stop eating and drinking after midnight the night before your scheduled surgery.

After TURP, you should plan on taking off 1 week, or more if you do heavy lifting.

Since TURP is a short operation lasting about an hour, you may be given a choice of having a regional, or spinal, anesthetic instead of a general anesthetic.

If you are having a regional anesthetic, you will not go to sleep. You will be asked to either turn to one side or sit up and bend forward as much as you can. This opens the space in your spine where a needle will be inserted. The skin on your lower mid-back is cleaned with an antiseptic solution and frozen with a small needle. After that, another needle is inserted into your lower back so the anesthetic can be delivered to your spinal cord to numb you from the waist down. You'll then lie on your back again and your anesthesiologist will test the feeling in your legs to see if the anesthetic has worked. You may also get some oxygen through a tube placed below your nose (**nasal prongs**).

Once the anesthesiologist has numbed you from the waist down or put you to sleep, your feet will be positioned into stirrups — what surgeons call the **lithotomy position** — in order to access the prostate through your penis. Antiseptic cleaning solution is applied to your penis and the area around it. Sterile drapes are then placed over the area where the surgery will take place. If you are having a spinal anesthetic, you won't be aware of what's going on during the procedure because there will be a barrier draped across your midsection, separating you from the surgical team.

Your surgeon will begin by inserting a telescopic device called a **resectoscope** into your urethra (see Figure 4–2). A fibre-optic video camera connected to the resectoscope allows the surgical team to watch the procedure on a monitor screen. You may be able to watch the screen if you receive a spinal anesthetic, but you don't have to watch if you don't want to. Once the resectoscope reaches your prostate, the obstructive tissue will be scraped out using **electrocautery**.

Electrocautery involves using a small probe charged with a high-energy electrical current to burn away the obstructive prostate tissue. This device seals off local blood vessels as it goes through tissue to minimize bleeding. A **grounding pad** will have been taped to your thigh before your surgery starts to prevent electrical shock.

Once your surgeon is satisfied with the amount of prostate tissue removed, the resectoscope is taken out and a catheter is inserted into your bladder via your urethra. See page 118 for more on catheters. After TURP, your bladder may be continuously flushed with slightly salty water (called a **saline solution**) to prevent the blood from clotting in your bladder. This is done by attaching a 3 litre bag of saline to one of your catheter ports. The catheter automatically drains your bladder through a second port into a urine bag. Once the procedure is over, you will be transferred to the **post-anesthetic care unit** (**PACU**) and your recovery can begin.

Figure 4-2: Transurethral Resection of the Prostate (TURP)

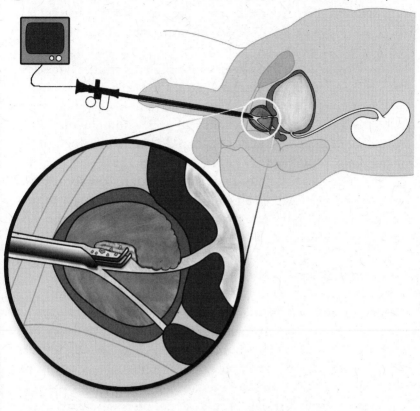

In TURP, *an instrument called a resectoscope is inserted into the prostate through the urethra. The resectoscope contains a tiny camera that allows the surgeon to watch the procedure on a video screen. An electrocautery probe uses an electrical current to destroy the enlarged prostate tissue.*

The Advantages of TURP

Studies have repeatedly shown that after TURP, patients don't have to urinate as often and their urinary flow is much stronger. The benefits of TURP are long-lasting, and the procedure reduces the chance that you'll need additional drug therapy. There's only a 1 in 20 chance that you'll need repeat surgery after

5 years. Repeat surgery becomes necessary if prostate tissue re-grows and obstructs the urinary passage, but this second procedure poses no greater risk than the original operation.

Recovery from TURP is fast because the procedure is done via the urethra, with no surgical **incision**. Once the catheter that was inserted in the urethra is removed after surgery, you should be able to urinate right away and will notice an immediate improvement in symptoms. You should be able to return to normal daily activities (light duties only) in as little as 1 week after the procedure, although complete healing usually takes about 6 weeks. TURP also generally causes few complications. Severe complications are extremely rare and the odds of not waking up are about 2 in 1000.

The Downsides of TURP
Although most men do well after TURP, 10 to 15 percent temporarily suffer a complication called urinary retention, in which they are unable to empty their bladder. A variety of factors contribute to this complication, such as an individual's overall health, whether he experienced acute urinary retention before the operation, and inflammation and bleeding caused by the surgery. If this happens to you, a catheter will be inserted into your bladder and removed several days later when you have healed properly. If there is excessive bleeding, the catheter will need to be irrigated with fluid in order to flush out any blood clots that may have formed.

If urinary retention occurs on a regular basis, a technique called **intermittent self-catheterization (ISC)** may help. The patient is taught to insert a catheter himself whenever urinary retention occurs, to relieve himself. For most men, this solution is only necessary for a short period and the bladder settles down in time. For a rare few, ISC may be needed indefinitely.

The opposite problem is urinary **incontinence**. Permanent urinary incontinence is very rare after TURP (fewer than 1 in 100 cases), and most men regain full bladder control. If you do experience incontinent symptoms, these are most likely to take the form of **stress incontinence** (loss of urine with coughing, laughing, exercising, and so on) or **urge incontinence** (involuntary loss of urine while suddenly feeling the need to urinate).

If this happens to you, your treatment options are exercises or medication. Exercises to help your sphincter muscles regain their strength are useful for stress incontinence. Urge incontinence can be treated with medications that relax the bladder to prevent uninhibited contractions that could cause leakage.

Another downside of TURP is that it can cause sexual dysfunction (erection difficulties) in about 1 in 25 patients. If this happens to you, bear in mind that many things can affect your erections, including fatigue after surgery and anxiety. There is unlikely to be a physical reason for **erectile dysfunction** after TURP, and the chances are good that things will improve with time. However, if you find that your erectile dysfunction does not improve, there are solutions—see page 183.

About 75 percent of patients will experience **retrograde ejaculation**, a harmless condition in which some (or all) of the ejaculate goes into the bladder, rather than out of the penis, during orgasm. This happens because the bladder no longer closes properly—either due to an injury to the bladder's sphincter muscle or damage to the nerves that control the sphincter. It is the most common side effect of TURP.

If this happens to you, you will notice that significantly less semen exits through your penis, and you may even experience a **dry climax** (orgasm without semen).

> ❗ [KEY POINT]
>
> **Deciding to treat BPH** depends
> primarily on how bothered you
> are by your urinary symptoms.
> Before you decide on surgery or
> medications, be sure to thoroughly
> discuss the risks and benefits of
> each with your urologist.

This condition is not dangerous, but it does affect your ability to father children. If you don't want any more children, retrograde ejaculation shouldn't concern you. If you still want to father children, however, mild problems can often be corrected with medications that improve muscle tone, such as ephedrine, pseudoephedrine or imipramine. Unfortunately, if your retrograde ejaculation is the result of severe damage to the nerves or muscle of your bladder's neck, then the condition is likely permanent. In this case, fertility specialists can rescue semen from your urine for in vitro fertilization, in which your partner's egg is fertilized with your sperm in the laboratory, then re-implanted into her uterus.

Minimally Invasive Treatments
Over the years the search has been on to find alternatives to TURP. Several minimally invasive procedures have been developed, some of which are still experimental, and others are available only at some hospitals or at private clinics. They include techniques to shrink or destroy the prostate tissue (**high-intensity focused ultrasound, transurethral electrovaporization, transurethral needle ablation**, and **hyperthermia**, or **thermotherapy**) and procedures to stretch and "prop open" the urethra (**transurethral balloon dilation** and **intraurethral stents**).

Two techniques that have gained popularity more rapidly than the others are **transurethral microwave thermotherapy (TUMT)** and **laser treatments**.

TUMT can be performed as a day procedure in the hospital or private clinic and uses microwaves to destroy the prostate tissue that is causing obstruction. Laser treatments "evaporate" the prostate gland internally or remove large pieces of tissue, without the bleeding and potential complications associated with standard TURP.

Two of the newest techniques are called **Green Light TURP** and the **Holmium laser** technique. Although these techniques have not been studied very extensively yet and their long-term benefits are still unknown, they do appear to genuinely improve symptoms and are more effective than alpha-blockers, one of the traditional medications for BPH (page 55). The downside of these procedures is that they may not be covered by healthcare plans, in which case you may be in for a bill of several thousand dollars.

Was Your TURP a Success?
You and your physician will decide whether your TURP has worked based on whether your urinary symptoms have improved. You may be asked to fill in another AUA symptom score (page 52) to measure how much your symptoms have improved, if at all.

Your physician may also choose to perform some of the same tests that you had before the operation, such as a uroflow test (page 52) or a post-void residual, for a "before and after" comparison. If you were having kidney problems due to obstructed urinary flow, he or she may also order blood tests to see if your kidney function has improved.

The surgery should have increased the strength of your urinary flow and reduced the amount of urinary frequency both during the day and during the night. Be prepared for the fact that frequency may not change right away. There may also be some urinary leakage for a few weeks while your tissues heal. If this continues for many months, consult your urologist.

BPH Treatment: Pros and Cons

There are many factors to consider when you're deciding what treatment is best for you. This quick reference chart may help.

	Advantages	Disadvantages
Watchful waiting	• No invasive procedures • No drugs • Up to half of BPH cases resolve by themselves	• A third of men experience progressive worsening of symptoms • Reserved for mild symptoms and low risk of urinary retention • Must avoid over-the-counter cold remedies • Water pills for hypertension worsen symptoms • Silent disease progression • Stones, infections, bleeding, impaired kidney function • 1 in 10 odds of acute urinary retention • 1 in 20 odds of surgery
Medications	• Safe and effective way to relax prostate sphincter muscle • Less urinary frequency and urgency	• Benefits are dependent on drug • Drugs may be required for a long time and some drugs are costly • Risk of side effects • Risk of urinary retention still exists

Continued...

	Advantages	Disadvantages
TURP	• Significantly less urinary frequency and urgency • Benefits long-lasting • No drugs • Low risk of repeat surgery • Quick recovery from a one-time event	• Discomfort, hospital stay, anesthetic • Rarely, acute urinary retention after surgery, requiring long-term catheterization • Erectile dysfunction in 1 in 25 • Incontinence in 1 in 100 • Retrograde ejaculation is common

What Happens Next?

As you regain your strength and energy after your TURP procedure, consider making some small lifestyle changes that will speed your recovery and help you regain your quality of life. Chapter 2 covers the benefits of diet for prostate health. Chapter 13 takes a detailed look at how to recapture your intimate life, while Chapter 14 gives some practical ways to benefit from the magical powers of exercise.

Chapter 5

what are your treatment options for prostate cancer?

What Happens in This Chapter
- What will happen if you do nothing?
- What are watchful waiting and active surveillance?
- What is radiotherapy?
- What is radical prostatectomy?
- The inside story on prostate cancer surgery
- What if treatment doesn't work?
- Pros and cons of other cancer options

If you are diagnosed with prostate cancer, your physician will use a whole raft of information, including your medical history, physical examinations, lab tests and imaging technology results, to come up with treatment recommendations that he or she thinks are best for you. However, the decision to proceed with treatment is yours. In some cases, test results are indisputable, the diagnosis certain and the benefits of treatment obvious. But sometimes things aren't so clear-cut. Understanding the benefits and drawbacks of your options may help you make this important decision.

How Much Time Do I Have?

If you have been diagnosed with prostate cancer, and it's confined to the prostate gland, your next big question is probably, "Now what?"

The worst thing you can do right now is panic. Do not rush into any immediate treatment decisions or feel you have to "settle your affairs." You are not in any immediate, life-threatening danger from your prostate cancer. Why not?

Thanks to many studies from the US, Canada and Europe, we now understand very well how prostate cancer develops if we do nothing—the so-called natural history of prostate cancer. Prostate cancer that is confined to the gland itself (i.e., hasn't spread) grows very slowly. There are exceptions to this, and fast-growing prostate tumours have been seen in a small minority of men, but in the majority of cases we measure prostate cancer growth by decades, not years. It can take 5, 10 or 20 years before prostate cancer spreads outside of the prostate gland.

How do we know this? A few years ago an increasing number of scientific papers reported that men who underwent autopsies after they had died from heart attacks or trauma were unexpectedly found to have prostate cancer. So, reasoned prostate cancer researchers, if the prostate cancer was "outliving" men, why should we bother to treat it? This led to further studies that observed what would happen over time when men were not actively treated after being diagnosed with prostate cancer.

Since prostate cancer takes its time to grow, and it tends to occur in older men who have other medical problems, it's much more likely that a man's life will be threatened by one of his conditions other than his prostate cancer. For example, a man who has had several heart attacks in the past and is then diagnosed with prostate cancer is much more likely to die from heart disease than from his prostate cancer. This means that many men, especially older men, are more likely to die *with* prostate cancer than *from* prostate cancer. On the other hand, a man who is diagnosed at the age of 50 and who is otherwise healthy *is* likely to experience problems with the progression of his prostate cancer.

However, not all prostate cancers have the same natural history. As we already mentioned, some are more aggressive (i.e., grow faster and are more likely to spread) than others. When you and your physician are making treatment decisions, it's obviously crucial to get some measure of how aggressive your cancer is likely to be. This is done using your Gleason score, your PSA and your tumour stage (see More Detail box the next page).

The bottom line is that if you have been diagnosed with prostate cancer nothing is likely to happen tomorrow, the next day, next month or even next year! You have lots of time to gather your information, learn about prostate cancer and decide what treatment is right for you. Don't be pushed into any decision that makes you feel uncomfortable.

Together with your specialist, you will need to consider two types of factors when you are making your decision:

- "Host" factors (i.e., you!): your age and your other medical conditions
- "Tumour" factors (i.e., your prostate cancer): Gleason score, PSA level and TNM stage

How Fast Will Your Prostate Cancer Progress?

One of the medical "crystal balls" that allows your physician to predict how fast your cancer will grow and spread is called the Gleason score (see also pages 41–42). In essence, the Gleason score is a measure of how aggressive your cancer cells look under the microscope. The Gleason score has been shown to be the best predictor of prostate cancer growth and progression for men whose prostate cancer is confined to the prostate gland. Studies from around the world have shown that men with a Gleason score of 8 to 10 have very aggressive cancer that will progress faster than men with a Gleason score of 6 or 7. If men with a Gleason score of 8 to 10 do not undergo treatment, 70 percent die from prostate cancer within 10 years, while only 10 percent of those with a Gleason score of 6 die over the same time period.

PSA levels and the stage of the tumour (described on pages 30–32 and 42–43) are also useful; a PSA level greater than 10 ng/mL or a tumour stage greater than T2 suggests that your cancer will be fairly aggressive.

Your specialist will take into account all three factors—the Gleason score, PSA level and tumour stage—to determine how aggressive your prostate cancer is. Although men generally have lots of time to make up their minds about what to do about their prostate cancer, sometimes the specialist concludes that the tumour is particularly aggressive and urgent treatment is necessary. Other times, the tumour may not be aggressive at all, and your specialist will do his or her best to be reassuring.

However, bear in mind that we still cannot predict with 100 percent certainty how your cancer will behave. Some low grade cancers (Gleason score 6) can be very aggressive, and some high grade cancers (Gleason score 9–10) may not be. Thus, it is important to realize that no one—not even your specialist—will have all the answers about your prostate cancer. Many researchers, including Dr Nam and his team, are hard at work to find new medical tests that are more accurate than our current methods.

With all these factors in mind, you and your specialist can then decide whether you should consider watchful waiting, radiation, surgery or medication-based treatment.

Prostate Cancer Treatment Options

For prostate cancer, there are currently four main options: a wait-and-see approach (watchful waiting or active surveillance), radiation therapy, surgical removal of the prostate (radical prostatectomy) and medication-based treatment. These options are summarized on page 95–96. If your physician recommends active treatment, it is worth realizing that radiation and surgery appear to be equally effective. So long as the cancer is confined to the prostate, the chances of a complete cure with either treatment are extremely good.

The Wait-and-See Approach

Option 1: Watchful Waiting
Watchful waiting involves having no treatment for your prostate cancer until you start having symptoms, at which time your physician will treat the symptoms only, usually with medication.

Watchful waiting can be very appealing for men who don't want any type of treatment for prostate cancer, because they avoid the potential side effects of cancer treatment such as urinary leakage (incontinence) or erection problems (erectile dysfunction). Watchful waiting is based on the assumption that you are more likely to die *with* prostate cancer and not *from* it.

Despite the appeal of "doing nothing," watchful waiting is really only an option for a select group of men. Men in their late 60s or older whose cancer appears less aggressive and men who are too ill from other causes to undergo treatment are the best candidates for watchful waiting. If your cancer has already started progressing, you will be advised to start curative treatment— radiotherapy or surgery—without delay.

> **!** [**KEY POINT**]
>
> **Watchful waiting is not a treatment.** It means doing nothing to "cure" your cancer, and simply treating symptoms as they arise. If you opt for watchful waiting and your cancer suddenly starts spreading between checkups, the goal of treatment is not to cure you but to treat your symptoms to make you feel better. Your oncologist will determine whether watchful waiting is an option for you, based on the characteristics of your own tumour.

If you opt for waiting, you'll need to have regular checkups. Your oncologist will do regular PSA (blood test) measurements and DRE (physical exam) checks to determine the status of your prostate cancer.

Option 2: Active Surveillance
Active surveillance is a new variation on the "wait-and-see" approach. As its name suggests, it involves monitoring your prostate cancer closely with regular PSA tests, DREs and prostate biopsies; at the first sign of prostate tumour growth and progression you would be offered radiation treatment or surgery. The key difference between active surveillance and watchful waiting is that treatment to cure your prostate cancer is still possible at the first sign of cancer progression—something

we refer to as "delayed curative therapy." The appeal of this approach is that someone may never need treatment; that is, he may turn out to have the type of prostate cancer that is slow growing—or not growing at all—and he would eventually die with the disease and not from it. The other major advantage of active surveillance is that, even if the man does eventually need treatment, at least he has several months or years free of treatment side effects.

What's the Catch?

The catch to either watchful waiting or active surveillance is that we don't have a test that can predict with 100 percent certainty the aggressiveness of a prostate tumour.

For a man who chooses watchful waiting, there are no absolute guarantees that his cancer will not progress. Some patients defy all the odds and turn out to have aggressive, rapidly progressing prostate cancer despite rosy results from the Gleason score, PSA level or stage. Even if a man chooses to play it safe and opts for active surveillance, there are no guarantees that his cancer will be curable once it starts to progress. Some recent studies have shown that men undergoing active surveillance who eventually require surgery to remove the prostate have higher rates of positive margins—cancer being left behind—which could reduce their chances of being cured. Further research is required to better understand what this means for patients who choose active surveillance.

> "I had come from the school where the doctor kind of recommends to you what to do. But in prostate cancer you have to make the decision for yourself. It's not made for you. You have to make your treatment decision based on your own lifestyle and what you can live with down the road."
>
> JIM

In both cases, you and your physician could have missed the window of opportunity for cure. Further research is being conducted to develop better markers for cancer aggressiveness. Until then, it is very important to understand the potential downsides before choosing watchful waiting or active surveillance.

Is It Possible to Cure Prostate Cancer?

You may, very reasonably, think that cancer treatments have been proven to cure cancer. Otherwise, why do them? It may come as a surprise, then, to realize that until recently many prostate cancer specialists did not believe that prostate cancer could be cured with the existing treatments. It was not until 2005 that a group of Scandinavian researchers demonstrated definitively that one treatment at least — prostate surgery — could save lives. The researchers from 14 cancer centres in Sweden, Finland and Iceland compared surgery to watchful waiting in a rigorous type of medical study where participants were randomly assigned to surgery or "do nothing" groups. The study found that, over 8 years, more men died of prostate cancer in the watchful waiting group than in the surgery group — almost twice as many, in fact. However, a more recent study from the US found slightly different results. The so-called PIVOT study did not find any difference between the watchful waiting or surgery groups when it came to saving lives, except in the men who had aggressive prostate cancer. Even so, it is hard to draw any definite conclusions from this; once the detailed results of the PIVOT study are released, the situation may be clearer.

The European study, at least, is great news for prostate surgery, but what about the alternative, radiation treatment? Unfortunately, no one has ever done a randomized clinical trial comparing watchful waiting with radiation for prostate cancer.

However, smaller studies suggest that radiation provides similar survival rates to surgery (see More Detail box), suggesting that it, too, is a "cure" for prostate cancer in many men.

Although surgery may be more obviously suited to some men than radiation, and vice versa, because they seem to be equally effective, often the choice of treatment is determined by the patient's own preferences.

Radiotherapy

Radiation therapy, or radiotherapy, works by using the energy from X-rays or particles to disrupt the DNA of the prostate cancer cells. This kills the cancer cells or "paralyzes" them, making them unable to divide and spread elsewhere. Using radiotherapy to treat cancer has been around for many years, but vast improvements in the planning and delivery systems have been made in the last two decades. Most studies of modern radiotherapy show that it is very effective in controlling cancer in most patients (see More Detail box).

The two main kinds of radiotherapy that are commonly used to treat prostate cancer are **external beam radiotherapy** and **brachytherapy**.

The main advantage of radiotherapy is that you are spared a major, invasive procedure. Side effects like sexual function and urinary incontinence are about the same as with surgery. External beam radiotherapy does not require any anesthetic, and although brachytherapy requires a general or regional anesthetic, this is a fairly minor outpatient procedure.

There are a number of factors to consider when you're trying to decide if radiotherapy is right for you. Radiation does have some other unpleasant side effects not seen with surgery, such as other urinary symptoms and irritation of the rectum. It can cause some patients to retain urine to the point where they can't empty their bladder at all—the condition called acute urinary retention. In addition, external beam radiation can require a significant time commitment (up to 2 months of treatment, 30 minutes every business day), which may be difficult to schedule if you're still working or live far from a treatment centre.

Radiation or Surgery? [MORE DETAIL]

Radiation and surgery appear to be equally effective at treating prostate cancer in certain patients and have similar 15-year survival rates. However, bear in mind that we don't know about survival beyond 15 years. The challenge in evaluating the newer radiation techniques is that because improvements are rapidly being introduced in the clinic, studies that are 15 years old use technology that is not in use today. Also, we still don't know if radiation works as well as surgery for more aggressive tumours.

External Beam Radiotherapy

This treatment approach involves directing radiation beams to the prostate using a device called a **linear accelerator**. Standard therapy consists of 10 to 15 minutes each day, 5 days a week, over a period of 6 to 8 weeks. You receive the radiation in daily, low-dose bursts to give the healthy tissue surrounding the prostate a chance to recuperate. Cancerous tissue doesn't repair itself as quickly as normal tissue, so over time the cancer cells cannot cope with the repeated bombardments and sustain so much damage that they are destroyed. However, the surrounding areas of normal tissue recover from the radiation damage.

Conformal Radiotherapy and IMRT

Three-dimensional conformal radiotherapy (3D-CRT), which has been in use for about 15 years in Canada, has added, literally, a new dimension to external beam radiotherapy. In this technique, multiple radiation beams (usually 4 to 6) are computer guided to deliver a custom-shaped dose of radiation to a three-dimensional target area, that is, the prostate and the areas where tiny prostate cancer cells may have spread. This means that higher doses can be delivered safely to the cancer while sparing the surrounding tissues, especially the rectum and the bladder. The computer software also allows your radiation oncologist to calculate the exact dose of radiation to be delivered to the target and the surrounding normal tissues, to keep side effects to a minimum.

A further refinement is an approach called **intensity-modulated radiotherapy (IMRT).** This technology goes one step further and allows the radiation oncologist to vary the number of radiation beams, as well as the dose and shape of individual beams. This allows him or her to conform the radiation dose even more tightly to the prostate, thus increasing your chances of a cure, with fewer unwanted effects on healthy tissue.

Image-Guided External Radiation

A technique that makes 3D-CRT or IMRT even more effective is called **image-guided radiotherapy (IGRT).** Traditionally, radiation is targeted at the prostate using skin tattoos that are placed with the help of a CT scan during a planning visit. The downside of this approach is that the prostate can move a few millimetres over time, so your radiation oncologist will add a 10 mm margin to the prostate "target," inevitably meaning that healthy tissues also get a dose of radiation. IGRT machines are smarter than that: they take an X-ray or CT of the pelvis just before the radiation treatment, verify the position of the prostate and then deliver the treatment. This shaves the "uncertainty margin" down considerably, sparing most normal tissue.

A combination of IGRT and IMRT is the most precise and accurate external radiation approach to date for your prostate cancer. It has huge advantages, allowing you to receive your treatment with fewer visits (sometimes as few as five), with fewer side effects and a greater chance of a cure.

Brachytherapy

There are two types of brachytherapy—permanent-seed brachytherapy and temporary-seed brachytherapy (high-dose rate [HDR] brachytherapy).

Approaches vary, but in most centres permanent-seed brachytherapy is reserved for patients with low-risk cancers— that is, a PSA below 10 ng/mL, a Gleason score of 6 or less, and a small or no nodule in the prostate (T1–T2) (see pages 36 and 38). For patients with higher-risk cancers, 1 to 2 HDR treatments are usually combined with a few weeks of external beam radiation.

Permanent seed brachytherapy is a one-time outpatient procedure that involves implanting about 80 to 100 radioactive "seeds," usually iodine or palladium, into the prostate through the skin between the anus and the base of the penis (the perineum). The seeds are positioned in the prostate using transrectal ultrasound guidance (see page 33) to lie approximately 5 mm (¼ inch) apart from each other. The radiation that comes from the seeds weakens significantly over a distance of only a few millimetres, so damage to nearby healthy tissues is limited, while the additive effect of numerous radioactive seeds results in a very high radiation dose delivered to the prostate. Although the seeds stay in the prostate permanently, their radioactivity fades away to nothing in 3 to 12 months.

The side effects of permanent-seed brachytherapy are similar to those experienced with external beam radiation but differ in key ways. First, the dominant short-term side effect is irritation to the bladder and urination tube (the urethra)—bowel irritation is relatively uncommon. Second, the intensity of the urinary side effects is much greater. Third, the side effects last longer. While the first month is the worst, it can take up to 6 months before you feel like you are back to normal.

HDR brachytherapy is similar in that freezing is given in your back (spinal anesthetic) to numb your pelvic area, and an ultrasound is used to guide the needle placement. In the case of HDR, small hollow tubes (about the diameter of the ink well of a ballpoint pen) are inserted through the perineum and into the prostate.

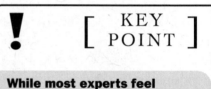

! [KEY POINT]

While most experts feel that the radiation of standard brachytherapy poses no danger to others, you will give off a very low dose of radiation, and you're advised not to hug infants and pregnant women for 2 months after seed implantation. By contrast, with HDR brachytherapy you are not radioactive after treatment.

Measurements are taken with the tubes in place, and a custom plan is generated. The tubes are then hooked up to the treatment machine that controls the insertion of a highly radioactive seed into the prostate, via the tubes. The treatment takes between 10 and 20 minutes. All the tubes are then removed. This may be preceded or followed by a few weeks of external radiation. Sometimes several of these HDR treatments are given over a few days, and the external radiation is not needed.

The side effects of HDR/external radiation are similar to those of external beam treatment.

Radical Prostatectomy (Surgery)

Surgery for prostate cancer is called radical prostatectomy. Making the decision to have surgery can be hard, even if it seems like the best and most obvious course of action. It involves complete removal of the prostate gland and the surrounding tissue, including the part of the bladder and structures called the seminal vesicles that are attached to the prostate.

There are different surgical options currently available in Canada—**open radical prostatectomy (ORP), laparoscopic radical prostatectomy (LRP) and robot-assisted laparoscopic**

> "I sailed through the radiation remarkably well. For the first 50 percent of the radiation, I had essentially zero side effects. In the second half of my program, I began to notice fatigue, which I had been warned about, and I began to notice that there was some looseness and some diarrhea, which affected me in the morning only. So I rescheduled my life so that I would tend to stay home in the morning. By noon, the diarrhea had passed, and the afternoon and evening were free to do whatever I chose to do."
>
> RON

radical prostatectomy (RALRP). There is a great deal of controversy surrounding the ideal surgery for prostate cancer, but it is important to note that regardless of the approach, the procedures are very similar. The open approach has the longest track record and in Canada remains the most commonly used.

In the traditional "open" technique, an incision 6 to 10 cm (3 to 4 inches) in length is made from your pubic bone to your belly button, and the surgeon removes your prostate "by hand" with standard surgical instruments. This procedure allows the surgeon to touch and feel the prostate, which at times is more important than the magnification offered with robotic approaches. Many surgeons say that until the robot can recreate the feeling of touch, it will never be superior to the open approach.

The second method is the laparoscopic approach—commonly called "keyhole" surgery. In this technique, about four to five small incisions are made through which long, telescopic instruments are inserted and guided by a video camera. The surgeon controls these long instruments from outside the body and surgically removes the prostate internally with the aid of the video camera.

The third, and newest, approach is the robot-assisted laparoscopic technique (see Figure 5–1). The main difference between this and the laparoscopic approach is that the instruments are not held by a surgeon, but by mechanical arms attached to a robot unit. This unit is then operated by the primary surgeon outside the operating room. The advantage of using robotic assistance is that the placement of the laparoscopic instruments is more precise. This is possible because the instruments are more intricate and have more "degrees of freedom," so they move more like a human hand inside the body. Robotic arms eliminate even the slightest hand tremors, and the instrument's "wrists" are quite versatile, allowing for greater maneuverability than human hands.

The operation, regardless of technique, takes approximately 2 to 3 hours, and you stay in the hospital for 1 to 2 days, depending on your surgeon. You are discharged with a catheter in place to drain your bladder; your surgeon removes the catheter about 1 to 2 weeks after the procedure. It usually takes about 4 to 6 weeks to recover fully. Robotic surgery is not for everyone, and your surgeon is the best person to tell you if you're a candidate for this type of operation. For a detailed description of radical prostatectomy, see Chapter 8.

Figure 5-1 The Robotic Procedure

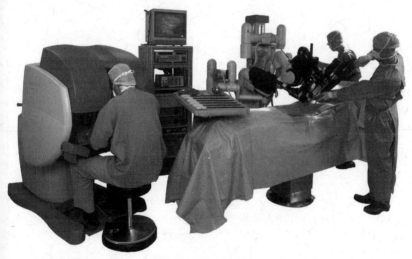

©2012 Intuitive Surgical, Inc.

Advantages of Surgery

One major advantage of surgery, regardless of which technique is used, is that we know it gives long-lasting control of prostate cancer. The open technique has been around for more

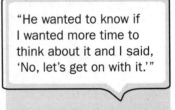

"He wanted to know if I wanted more time to think about it and I said, 'No, let's get on with it.'"

RAY

than 50 years, and the procedure itself has been done for over 100 years—much longer than any other prostate cancer treatment. Repeated studies have shown that a high percentage of patients who have radical prostatectomy have excellent long-term survival (20 years or more).

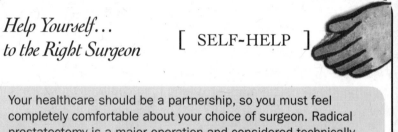

Help Yourself...
to the Right Surgeon   [SELF-HELP]

Your healthcare should be a partnership, so you must feel completely comfortable about your choice of surgeon. Radical prostatectomy is a major operation and considered technically difficult. A study published in the prestigious *New England Journal of Medicine* showed that patients suffered fewer complications when their surgeon had performed the procedure often (at least 33 times per year). The same is true if you choose laparoscopic or robotic surgery. It takes some time to do these techniques well. Some studies have shown that it might take 50 to 100 procedures before the surgeon becomes proficient.

Surgeon experience is often studied in what are called "volume-outcome analyses" and "evaluation of learning curves." Simply put, these kinds of analyses measure how the surgeon improves at performing the surgery as he or she does more of them.

Keep in mind that urologists are qualified to perform a wide variety of different surgical procedures and that radical prostatectomy is only one of many. Don't be shy. It's up to you to ask whether this is a procedure that your urologist performs frequently.

The other major advantage is that when the whole prostate gland is removed, a pathologist can examine the tumour in detail to see whether the cancer was confined to the prostate gland and all of the cancer was removed. With this information, your oncologist can determine if further treatment is needed.

86

Sometimes, radiation may be required after the surgery to get better control of the cancer. Other times, hormone medications alone, or together with radiation therapy, are used. Having a detailed examination of exactly how far the cancer has spread will help your oncologist to make these decisions. On the other hand, knowing that the cancer was completely confined within the prostate can provide peace of mind.

Nerve Sparing and Nerve Grafting [MORE DETAIL]

Radical prostatectomy is now a more attractive option than it once was, with the arrival of improved techniques for sparing the nerves that control erections and urination. You should discuss **nerve-sparing** techniques with your surgeon, although he or she will make the final decision on what is practical during the actual surgery, based on how extensive your cancer is.

When both nerves that control erections are spared, the probability for having erections after surgery is high—between 60 and 80 percent. However, bear in mind that this is an average. If you have other medical conditions that affect erections, such as diabetes, depression or cardiovascular disease, the odds will be lower.

Nerve grafting is a new technique reserved for men who are sexually active and whose nerves cannot be spared due to the stage of their cancer. Early results seemed encouraging, but longer-term results were less inspiring, so although the procedure is available in a few hospitals, it is not yet widely practiced. Where nerve grafting is performed, results vary, so you and your surgeon should discuss whether this approach is right for you.

Disadvantages of Surgery

The downside of surgery is that it is a major operation and, like all surgeries, has risks associated with it. Bear in mind that the risks given below are averages, and, depending on your health, your own risks may be much lower (or higher). Your physician should discuss these risks with you.

Blood loss is the first downside to consider (see also page 108). If your surgeon is experienced, your chance of requiring a blood transfusion, on average, is about 1 to 10 percent. Laparoscopic/robotic surgery may be associated with less blood loss, most likely due to two reasons: (1) the surgeon has a better view, allowing him or her to better identify your blood vessels, and (2) the procedure itself involves introduction of carbon dioxide, which reduces bleeding. Most centres will cite a less than one unit blood loss, which is what you would usually give to the Canadian Red Cross if donating blood. This means that a blood transfusion is not usually required. Ask your surgeon what his or her transfusion record is.

The risk of death during radical prostatectomy is low, less than 0.5 percent. About 1 in 100 patients suffer a heart attack, blood clots in the veins (which in rare cases move to the lungs) or similar "cardiovascular" problems.

Because the prostate is quite close to the rectum and held in place by connective tissue, there's also a remote chance that the rectum could be injured. This complication is repaired on the spot and usually does not affect recovery time.

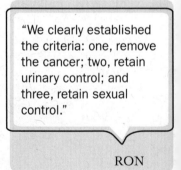

"We clearly established the criteria: one, remove the cancer; two, retain urinary control; and three, retain sexual control."

RON

Another problem that might develop after surgery is excessive scar tissue formation where the bladder is reconnected to the urethra. This condition is called a **bladder neck stricture** and occurs in 1 to 10 percent of patients. A procedure done in your doctor's office, involving a small incision into the stricture, easily corrects this complication.

Erectile dysfunction is one of the most feared side effects of prostatectomy. Many men will experience at least temporary problems with erections after their surgery, although for most this is not permanent. If your erection nerves are spared you are less likely to have problems (see More Detail box on page 87). You are also more likely to have good erections after surgery if you had good erections beforehand. Some medications, such as those for high blood pressure or heart disease, can also affect your ability to achieve an erection, and age can make a difference: the younger you are, the higher the probability that you will retain your erectile function. On the other hand, if one or more erection nerves had to be removed because the cancer had spread beyond the prostate, the likelihood of achieving erections after surgery will be lower. You are also less likely to have good erectile function after surgery if you have certain medical conditions, such as diabetes, depression or coronary artery disease. For a detailed discussion of sex after prostate surgery, see Chapter 13.

Incontinence is another potential disadvantage of prostatectomy that you should consider. Most men will experience at least temporary problems with incontinence after

> **!** **[KEY POINT]**
>
> **Whatever turns you on now** will turn you on after your surgery. It is important to realize that, although surgery can affect your ability to have an erection, it does not affect any other aspect of your sexuality. Even if you cannot get an erection at first, you can still get aroused, still feel sensation and still have an orgasm. The reason for this is that surgery rarely affects the nerves that control sensation, which are more widely spread than the erection nerves.

radical prostatectomy, but the odds of having permanent urinary control problems have fallen significantly in recent years with new techniques to prevent damage to the urethra, and are now only about 1 in 100. The vast majority of men have complete urinary control once they recover from surgery, although a few, 1 to 10 percent, will report mild leakage during coughing or laughing (called stress incontinence).

Development of an **incisional hernia** is uncommon, regardless of surgical option, but you should be aware that it can occur. It is caused by stress placed on the surgical site. To help avoid this, it is recommended that you avoid heavy lifting—anything greater than 5 kilograms (about 10 pounds)—or straining the abdominal muscles for 6 weeks after surgery.

Finally, recovery from prostatectomy can be uncomfortable. Most men will experience a bruised and swollen scrotum and/or penis after surgery because of blood pooling below the surgical site. Like any bruise, this may take a few weeks to settle down. For this reason, underwear such as briefs are recommended, as boxers do not support the scrotum. Another reason for discomfort after surgery is that you will have to live with a catheter coming out of your bladder and through your penis for about 1 to 2 weeks.

Comparing Surgeries and Outcomes

Recent studies have shown that laparoscopic surgery, robot-assisted laparoscopic surgery and the traditional open technique are very similar when it comes to curing prostate cancer. However, there has never been a randomized trial (a study where patients are randomly assigned to have one type of surgery or the other) to determine which procedure is better. In other diseases, laparoscopic and robotic surgeries are associated with less pain after surgery and a faster recovery, but in prostate cancer it's still not certain that laparoscopic or robotic surgeries are better.

Patient expectations also come into play when deciding which type of surgery is better. Patients who choose laparoscopy often have unrealistically high hopes about these "minimally invasive" procedures—hopes that are doubly dashed when urinary and sexual function don't fully return to normal afterward.

From a healthcare system perspective, LRP and RALRP are more costly procedures. Unlike the US, only a few hospitals across Canada offer these two procedures.

The table below compares the procedures in terms of outcomes.

Considerations when undergoing prostate cancer surgery	Open radical prostatectomy	Laparoscopic and robot-assisted laparoscopic radical prostatectomy
Blood loss	1–10%	1–5 %
Death	Less than 0.5%	Same
Rectal injury	Negligible	Same
Urethral stricture	2–10%	1–3%
Stress incontinence	1–10%	Same
Erectile function	Approximately 60–80% return of function if bilateral nerve sparing	Same
Length of stay in hospital	1–2 days	Same
Resume usual activities	6 weeks	Same
Pain management	Dependent on the institution	Same

When considering a variety of aspects of surgery, you'll notice that the open and laparoscopic/robotic approaches are quite similar. Ultimately, your surgeon will discuss the best technique with you, based on the characteristics of your prostate cancer.

What If My Surgery or Radiation Doesn't Work?

A common question among patients considering surgery or radiation is, what happens if treatment fails? If you have surgery and the cancer returns, can you still have radiation? Or, if you have radiation and the cancer returns, can you have surgery?

The first thing to say is that your decision to have surgery or radiation should not depend on these kinds of "what if" scenarios. Make the best choice now and rely on your primary treatment, which has a very good chance of curing you.

That said, it is worth bearing in mind that radiation can be used if the cancer returns after surgery, but surgery can be very challenging after radiation failure. The reason for this is that a radiation-damaged prostate is very difficult to remove without damaging structures such as the rectum and bladder. Studies also show that urinary problems, such as incontinence and blockage, are much more likely after such "salvage" surgery. Nonetheless, if you are in this position, don't despair. With an experienced surgeon, salvage radical prostatectomy has proven safe and effective in many men who have failed radiation treatment. For more on salvage treatments, see page 154.

Drug Therapy

Drug treatment is usually reserved for men who cannot have surgery or radiotherapy. For example, men whose prostate cancer has already metastasized (i.e., spread to other organs) beyond the prostate gland, or who have other medical conditions that rule out surgery or radiation. Drugs are also helpful after surgery or radiation as a preventive measure for very aggressive cancers or as a treatment if the cancer returns.

Hormone Treatments

About 50 years ago Charles Huggins, an American urologist, discovered that prostate cancer grows in response to male hormones (**androgens**), of which testosterone is the most important. This discovery not only meant a Nobel prize for Dr Huggins, but also an effective alternative treatment for men with prostate cancer. There is now a wide range of drug treatments that shrink prostate cancer by interfering with testosterone.

The huge advantage of these medications for prostate cancer, compared with "conventional" **chemotherapy**, is that hormonal approaches target only testosterone. They do not affect other organs or body systems — so they are generally well tolerated, regardless of whether you have other illnesses.

The downside of these drugs is that lack of testosterone can itself cause side effects, which you have to weigh against their life-saving effects. You may feel tired and fragile due to loss of muscle strength. Osteoporosis (brittle bones) and anemia are also long-term risks. Loss of **libido** and sexual function, and hot flashes, are also common complaints.

LHRH Agonists
Luteinizing hormone-releasing hormone (LHRH) agonists are artificial versions of a natural hormone called luteinizing hormone-releasing hormone. They work by stimulating the pituitary gland, a small gland tucked underneath the brain, to produce a hormone called luteinizing hormone (LH). At first this stimulates the testicles to produce more testosterone, but then a complex feedback mechanism kicks in; it dampens down LH production, and then testosterone levels start to fall. Within about 3 weeks, testosterone levels in the body become almost undetectable and stay that way as long as therapy is continued.

LHRH agonists need to be given by injection under your skin or into a muscle every 1 to 4 months. Your oncologist administers them. Four LHRH agonists are currently available in Canada: leuprolide (Eligard, Lupron and Trelstar) and goserelin (Zoladex).

LHRH Antagonists

This type of drug has recently become available in the US and Canada. Instead of initially stimulating the pituitary gland, **LHRH antagonists** do the opposite and immediately suppress it, which in turn tells the testicles to produce less testosterone. LHRH antagonists work faster than LHRH agonists to reduce testosterone levels. They also reduce other hormone levels, which may help them work better than LHRH agonists, but further research is needed in this area.

LHRH antagonists are injected under your skin every month. One LHRH antagonist is available in Canada: degarelix (Firmagon).

Antiandrogens

Another approach is to leave testosterone blood levels unchanged but prevent testosterone from "switching on" the prostate cancer cells. **Antiandrogen** medications do this by blocking testosterone at the level of the prostate cancer cells. Like a false key in the ignition, they block the testosterone receptors on the outside of prostate cancer cells, preventing the testosterone "key" from entering. These drugs are used together with LHRH agonists to help suppress the initial surge of testosterone. They can also be used to help LHRH agonists during treatment. Antiandrogens are usually not used alone.

Two antiandrogens are currently available in Canada: bicalutamide (Casodex) and flutamide (Euflex), but bicalutamide is often the preferred drug since it is associated with fewer side effects.

> "They were all telling me how young I was and how I can't just wait around and let this thing get the better of me. I should be getting the better of it."
>
> JIM

Chemotherapy

Some cases of advanced prostate cancer become resistant to hormone therapy, and the cancer starts to grow and progress despite this treatment. In this case, new chemotherapy agents such as docetaxel (Taxotere) are used. Taxotere-based chemotherapy has revolutionized the treatment for patients with so-called **hormone-refractory prostate cancer**. Studies have shown that it can dramatically improve quality of life and survival, which has never been shown before with chemotherapy regimens in prostate cancer.

Prostate Cancer Treatment—Pros and Cons

Treatment	Advantages	Disadvantages
Wait-and-see (watchful waiting or active surveillance)	• No invasive procedures • No drugs	• Side effects: – None • Higher risk of mestastases (cancer spreading) compared with surgery • Not a cure

Radiation	• Very effective in controlling cancer in most patients
	• Beam therapy is noninvasive
	• Beam therapy doesn't require anesthesia
	• Less chance of erectile problems compared with surgery
		• Side effects:
		  – Urinary incontinence
		  – Urinary retention
		  – Erectile dysfunction
		  – Radiation cystitis
		  – Rectal bleeding
		  – Proctitis
		  – Secondary cancers
		  – Mild fatigue very common
		• Beam therapy takes up to 8 weeks, 15 minutes a day, 5 days a week
		• Anesthesia necessary with brachytherapy
		• Impotence rates similar to surgery
		• Can't check out the tumour because it's left in place
		• Surgery after radiation often not possible

Continued...

Treatment	Advantages	Disadvantages
Surgery (open, LRP and RALRP)	• Excellent long-term survival for many men • One operation, lasting from 90 to 180 minutes • Pathology report on whole prostate • Greater certainty about cancer spread • Can have radiation after surgery	• Side effects: – Urinary incontinence – Erectile dysfunction – Scar tissue buildup leading to urinary difficulty – Rectal injury (rare) • Invasive procedure • Potential for blood loss, usually does not require transfusion • General anesthesia necessary • Catheter for about 2 weeks • Usually 6 weeks to recover fully • At least temporary urinary incontinence and erectile dysfunction
Hormone treatments	• May improve survival • Non-surgical option • Effective alternative if surgery or radiation not possible • Effective prevention for aggressive cancers	• Side effects: – Osteoporosis – Heart disease – Hot flashes – Loss of libido – Sexual dysfunction – Fatigue, weakness • Not a cure • LHRH agonists need to be injected every 1 to 4 months

Management of Side Effects

Because we are all different, we respond differently to treatment. Individual variability is normal in the type and severity of side effects for any given treatment option. It is important that you document your side effects and discuss them with your healthcare team. They will know how to best manage your side effects and may also suggest techniques or resources to help you.

What Treatment Is Right for Me?

Unfortunately, as previously discussed, despite many studies it is still not possible to say with certainty which treatment is best for patients with prostate cancer. Ultimately, it becomes a personal decision for the patient and his loved ones. Specialists will be able to provide important information about each treatment choice, but keep in mind that every specialist has his or her own bias about what the right treatment is. In general, surgeons will lean toward surgery, and radiation oncologists will lean toward radiation. Therefore, it is important for you to speak with surgeons and radiation oncologists in order to get a balanced opinion and make an informed decision about treatment.

What Happens Next?

If you and your physician decide to go ahead with surgery, the next chapter will help get you ready to take this important step to improving your health. If you decide that surgery isn't right for you, skip to Chapter 12 to find out how you can improve your long-term quality of life. You may also want to read Chapter 16 if you're curious to learn more about some of the medications you might be taking.

Chapter 6

getting ready for your surgery

What Happens in This Chapter
- Psyching up for surgery
- Pre-surgery arrangements
- The pre-admission clinic
- Giving consent
- Bowel preparation
- Blood transfusion options

You've weighed your options carefully and made a hard decision, but your work doesn't end there. Reading up on your procedure will help you to get organized and feel more prepared for your operation. Don't be afraid to ask lots of questions so that you're ready to face the challenge of what lies ahead. Once you've passed the physical exam at the pre-admission clinic, the next step is the surgery itself.

Getting Mentally Prepared

Well, here you are—in line for surgery. Although you'd probably rather get the operation over and done with quickly, you may have to wait a while before it's your turn. Not only will the hospital have to schedule surgery, but your surgeon may also prefer to wait at least 6 to 8 weeks after your biopsy to allow any swelling around the prostate to go down. Swelling might make it technically difficult to remove your prostate. However, this period of waiting provides a great opportunity to get organized for the weeks ahead.

Get a Helping Hand

We know—you're tough and can handle a lot. But part of being strong is knowing when to accept help: this is one of those times. You'll need a trusted companion to accompany you to your appointments. This person can be your partner, a close friend or other family member. It's important to remember that you need to feel comfortable with the person who is coming with you, as many intimate details will be discussed at your appointments. The right person can offer moral support, help the time pass in the waiting room and, most importantly, provide a second set of ears. Often, while you're engaged in the unfamiliar business of hospital protocols, you may miss important details or forget to ask a question you had in mind. Your companion can fill in the gaps and later confirm your own impressions of what was said at an appointment.

Once you've checked that your companion is available to come with you, it's important that you learn all you can about your procedure. Many people find that knowing more makes them less afraid of what's to come and helps them prepare for a more effective recovery. If you're reading this book, you've already started taking the next important step to psyching up for surgery. Take this time to learn and increase your knowledge about your prostate cancer and its treatment.

Talking with other men who have undergone prostate surgery will confirm what you have learned from us and may help to reassure you further. If you have prostate cancer, you may also want to consider joining a prostate support group in your area; ask the local cancer society, or your community or university hospital.

Ask Questions

It's also important to ask questions—lots of questions. There is no such thing as a dumb question when it comes to your health. Getting the answers you feel you need will give you more control over what's happening. While you're asking questions, feel free to verbalize your fears. It's normal to feel anxious about your surgery, and talking about your worries can make you less fearful.

Take Notes

Another suggestion is to take notes. You'll be better prepared for appointments and tests if you keep track of important dates, contacts and medical information. We've included a diary section at the end of this book to help you create your own personal medical history. Aside from jotting down your various appointments, tests and treatments, be sure to include any other health conditions you may currently have and all the medications (herbal, prescription and non-prescription) that you are taking. Making a note of your allergies and family history of serious illnesses is also helpful. Pull together your health insurance papers and keep them with your journal; you'll need them to find out what expenses are covered by your insurance plan.

Here are some questions that you may want to ask before your surgery:

- How might this surgery help me?
- What might happen if I don't have it?
- What are the alternatives?
- How might the surgery affect my sex life?
- Is it possible to spare my nerves for erections?
- Is it possible to perform nerve grafting if nerves have to be removed?
- Will I have problems with urination after my surgery?
- What can I do to reduce my risk of having a blood transfusion?
- What other risks are there?
- What should I bring with me to the hospital?
- How long will I be in the hospital?
- How long should I plan to take off work?
- Will I be in any pain after the surgery?

If you have had previous medical tests for any related or unrelated medical conditions, try to get a copy of your file from your family physician and bring it with you to your pre-admission appointment. Although your healthcare team will usually try to order these reports, it may be helpful if you already have them with you.

After your pre-admission appointment, it is a good idea to visit the department where you will be checking in on the morning of your surgery. Each hospital will have its own systems and areas for patient check-in, and knowing where you're going on the morning of the surgery will be a real help in reducing your anxiety.

Pre-surgery Arrangements

The time after your surgery is when you'll need help the most. Getting enough rest during your recovery is important for preventing complications and ensuring that you feel better faster. If you are responsible for household duties, it's a good idea to stock up on groceries and fill the freezer before your surgery. You should also arrange for friends or family to come and cut the grass or shovel snow for a few weeks after you come out of hospital.

After a radical prostatectomy, regardless of surgical technique, you may need 3 to 6 weeks off work, depending on how strenuous your job is and how much heavy lifting is involved. If you have a very sedentary office job where you control your own hours, you may be able to return as early as 3 weeks. But even in this case, you should not engage in any activity more strenuous than walking for 6 weeks, after which you can gradually increase your activity level. Although your body has amazing healing capabilities, remember, it can only do so many things at once. Returning to work too quickly may mean that healing takes a back seat to the stresses of work. You will still heal but it may take longer, especially for continence and erectile function. You should also avoid riding a bicycle for 2 to 3 months after surgery—many men say the pressure in the perineal area makes it difficult to sit comfortably on a bike seat.

"Don't be afraid to ask questions of your doctor. If your doctor is evasive or is not able or willing to answer your question then you simply run, don't walk, to the nearest exit and find yourself a physician that is. Don't be embarrassed to look for a second opinion.... A urologist is a surgeon by background and will offer surgery where it might be applicable, but don't think that it's the only answer."

RON

The Pre-admission Clinic

Arguably, operating rooms are among the most exclusive and valuable pieces of real estate in Canada, so it's not surprising that you have to fill out a lot of paperwork and undergo tests to qualify for entry. This all happens at the pre-admission clinic. It's an opportunity to get through the administration, have some tests and learn about what's to come. You'll meet a nurse, and possibly an anesthesiologist, and get answers to your questions. If there's one day you should really have this book and your companion with you, it's the day of the pre-admission clinic.

First up is paperwork such as hospital registration and a health insurance check. Then you go to the clinic where administrative staff will review general information with you, such as what wing and what floor of the hospital you'll be admitted to on the day of surgery, visiting hours and the location of waiting rooms, the cafeteria and parking. You might want to ask your companion to take notes for your journal, so you can focus your attention on the flood of details.

The nurse will check if you use assistive devices, such as a walker, a brace or a cane. If you live alone, he or she will discuss how you will manage everyday tasks at home after your surgery.

In most hospitals, before you are admitted you will be tested for bugs called methicillin-resistant *Staphylococcus aureus* (MRSA) and vancomycin-resistant *Enterococcus* (VRE). *Staphylococcus aureus* is a bacterium normally found on the skin and inside the nasal passages of healthy people. Some kinds—known as MRSA—have developed resistance to many of the commonly used antibiotics. Enterococci are bacteria normally found in your bowel. VRE have developed a resistance to some or all antibiotics commonly used to treat enterococcal infections.

If you are healthy, these two types of bacteria do not usually pose a problem, but for those whose immune resistance is low, they can be quite a serious health concern. If you are carrying MRSA you will receive a special treatment to clear your system of the bacteria. There is no special treatment for VRE.

Next will come the usual array of tests that all people facing surgery must undergo: an electrocardiogram (ECG) to gauge heart function, a chest X-ray to check your lungs, and blood tests. The blood tests measure how well your blood carries oxygen (**hemoglobin**), your body maintains normal fluid balance (**electrolytes**) and your kidneys remove waste (**creatinine**). If you have heart problems, diabetes or another ongoing health problem, you may be examined by another physician, such as a general internist. Be sure to tell your physician about *all* the medications you are taking, including over-the-counter drugs, such as vitamin E or anti-inflammatories (see Key Point on following page). It is particularly important to tell your surgeon and anesthesiologist if you are taking any anti-inflammatory medication such as ASA, or anticoagulant medication (e.g., Coumadin or Fragmin). If you are taking an anticoagulant you will either be instructed to stop the medication or arrangements will be made to reverse the effects of medication.

Meeting Your Anesthesiologist

Once you know you are having prostate surgery, you may meet with an anesthesiologist to discuss the anesthetics he or she may use. If you've had surgery before, tell him or her about any past complications with anesthetics—or if anyone in your family has ever had problems with anesthetics—including a rare syndrome called **malignant hyperthermia**. This condition involves a rapid spike in temperature (sometimes exceeding 40°C or 105°F) accompanied by severe muscle spasms.

Most patients will meet with their anesthesiologist only once before their surgery, usually in the holding area just before the operation. Depending on medical history, some patients may have an appointment to meet with the anesthesiologist during the pre-admission appointment. In either case, it's a good idea to come prepared, with a complete medical history, a description of all of your symptoms and any questions you might have. Having a complete record of your medical information and copies of past tests will help him or her give you more accurate information.

! **[KEY POINT]**

Vitamin E and anti-inflammatory drugs decrease the ability of your blood to clot and can cause excessive bleeding during surgery. The decision about whether you stop or continue your anti-inflammatory drugs will depend on the reasons why you are on them. Your doctor will look at the risks and benefits to see if it is safer for you to be on or off the medication. If you have to temporarily get off these drugs, you'll be asked to stop 10 days before your operation.

Common anti-inflammatory products include:

Acetylsalicylic acid (ASA)	Entrophen (ASA)
Advil (ibuprofen)	Ibuprofen
Aspirin (ASA)	Midol (contains ASA)
Alka-Seltzer (contains ASA)	Novasen (ASA)
Anaprox (naproxen)	Pepto-Bismol (contains ASA)
Celebrex (celecoxib)	Robaxisal (ASA)
Dristan (may contain ibuprofen)	

Consent

You make decisions to take risks every day of your life. Some kind of risk is involved when you cross a road, place a bet on a horse, drive your car or board an airplane. However, when you go into the hospital to have surgery, the risk you take feels different because you are allowing somebody else, usually a doctor, to make decisions for you. Nonetheless, it is a risk just like in many other parts of life.

Although the doctor will be acting in your best interest, it is still important that you understand exactly what you are giving your permission for, or consent to. You are therefore entitled to know what is going to happen to you, why the procedure is needed and what the risks are.

"It's tough to make your decision about how you're going to tackle it—what treatment you're going to go with and why. Once you've made all of those decisions, it's tough waiting for it to take place. I was very anxious; I was nine jumps ahead of the stick. I wasn't focusing on my work, hardly anything. Just wondering."

JIM

You may be asked for consent for your prostate surgery as soon as you agree to have the operation, in a pre-admission clinic, or on the day of your procedure. It is important that you read the consent form and understand what it is you are signing. Take a few moments to read through it, and, if there is enough time, you can take the form home and bring it back on the day of your procedure. If you are worried about any part of the procedure, or you feel you have not received a clear answer on anything, now is the time to say so.

Eating and Drinking Before Surgery

Most surgeons require that you stop eating solid food 24 hours before your surgery and restrict yourself to clear fluids such as ginger ale, tea, clear broth, popsicles, Jell-O and juice without pulp until midnight before surgery. After midnight, you should not eat or drink anything at all. Each centre has varying degrees of restrictions with timelines for when to stop all intake. Your healthcare team will inform you of exactly what these restrictions are.

Consent **[MORE DETAIL]**

There are three types of consent:

Implied consent—usually reserved for minor procedures such as blood tests or having a tongue depressor put into your mouth. In these cases, you non-verbally comply by sticking your arm out or opening your mouth.

Verbal consent—can be used in an emergency situation, when there is no time to obtain a signature on a consent form.

Written consent—needed before medical procedures that require an anesthetic because you will be given drugs that make you drowsy or put you to sleep. Since you will not be able to give your consent to your physician during your procedure, written consent—a legally binding document—is needed before the operation.

Preparations for Surgery

Bowel Prep

There's a small chance that your rectum might be injured during prostate surgery, so to be on the safe side, most hospitals will require you to empty your bowels to reduce the risk of septic infection. This is done by taking a laxative or giving yourself an enema the night before the operation.

Aside from reducing the infection risk, there's another benefit to bowel prep. Because the anesthetics and narcotics administered during surgery tend to slow down your intestinal tract, empty bowels mean you won't feel too bloated or constipated in the days following your procedure. More importantly, you won't have to strain to have a bowel movement, which can be especially uncomfortable if you have an abdominal incision. The straining may also cause a bladder spasm or a small amount of bleeding from around the catheter area. This is usually nothing to worry about, but keeping the bowel movements soft will avoid these uncomfortable side effects.

Blood Transfusions

The chances of requiring a blood transfusion during radical prostatectomy have fallen dramatically in recent years. If your physicians think you might need a blood transfusion, they will carefully consider its risks and benefits. The following are important principles of blood conservation, some of which need to be planned 4 to 6 weeks in advance of your surgery. You can also obtain reliable information on blood conservation from Canadian Blood Services (www.bloodservices.ca).

Why Is a Transfusion Needed?

If you lose blood during your surgery, your hemoglobin level may fall and your body tissues may have trouble getting enough oxygen. This is called **anemia** and can lead to fatigue, a slow recovery and impaired healing. A blood transfusion replenishes your hemoglobin to prevent this.

The amount of blood you lose depends on a number of factors, including the size of your prostate gland (there is more bleeding with a large gland) or other factors that may affect your health, such as your weight.

How Risky Is a Blood Transfusion?

In Canada, a blood transfusion has never been safer. Blood is collected from healthy volunteers by Canadian Blood Services or Héma-Québec and tested for a wide range of viruses, including hepatitis B and C, and HIV. The risk of becoming infected with one of these viruses is now quite small (see Key Point box on page 111). Other common risks of blood transfusions are fever and itchiness, which occur in around 1 in 100 people and are easily treated. Rejection reaction (**hemolytic reaction**), caused by the incompatibility of the two blood types or your immune system responding to the donor blood, also occurs in around 1 in 500,000 people. It is mostly prevented by a special blood test before your surgery, called **cross-matching**.

What Are Your Chances of a Transfusion?

Only about 1 to 10 percent of patients undergoing traditional radical prostatectomy need a blood transfusion after surgery. With laparoscopic and robotic techniques the rate is even lower, at 1 to 5 percent. The single most important factor in needing a transfusion after surgery is anemia before surgery. This is one of the reasons your blood is tested before your prostate surgery, so that you and your physician can correct your anemia before you have your procedure.

Blood Conservation Strategies
Identifying and Treating Anemia
Treating anemia before surgery is one of the most important things you and your physician can do to reduce the chances of a blood transfusion. If your blood tests before surgery show that your hemoglobin is low, your physician may prescribe iron tablets, vitamins (e.g., B12 or folate) or injections of a hormone called **erythropoietin**. Erythropoietin is naturally secreted by the kidneys to stimulate the body to make more red blood cells and a synthetic version (epoetin alfa [Eprex] or darbepoetin alfa [Aranesp]) will gradually correct your anemia by increasing the number of red blood cells in your body.

Donation of Your Own Blood
Donating your own blood, or **autologous blood donation (ABD)**, is sometimes an option for reducing your anxiety about receiving someone else's blood. It involves coming to the clinic or hospital 2 or 3 times before your surgery to donate one unit of blood at a time. Your blood is stored in the blood bank and reserved for your use for up to 35 days. If your stored blood is not used by you, it is discarded.

A relatively new ABD program called ALYX is available in some hospitals. This technique can remove 2 units of blood at the same time and does not require frequent visits. It is usually done 2 weeks before your surgery. However, not all hospitals offer this service.

You should talk to your physician at least 4 weeks before your surgery if you are interested in blood banking. Bear in mind it may not be available at your hospital, particularly if blood loss rates and transfusion rates are very low, or if your surgeon doesn't recommend it for your operation because your risk of a blood transfusion is very low.

Pre-donating blood may seem an attractive option since it reduces the risk that you will need donor blood, but it does have a number of disadvantages, and you and your physician should weigh these carefully against its benefits. Despite careful storage and handling of your pre-donated blood, there is a (small) risk that it could become infected with bacteria that will be passed on to you. There is also the small risk of clerical error, so you could end up receiving the wrong blood—equivalent to having a regular blood transfusion. The most important downside to pre-donating your own blood is that it may cause anemia before surgery, and if you do not receive your blood back this may make you anemic after surgery. Finally, bear in mind that despite having banked your own blood you may still receive a regular transfusion for medical reasons.

Planning Ahead

If you are anemic, remember that taking your iron tablets as prescribed and eating an iron-rich diet may help reduce the risk of having a blood transfusion. Iron-rich foods include

> **!** **[KEY POINT]**
>
> **Donor blood transfusions** are potentially life-saving and have never been safer. The risk of HIV infection from donated blood in Canada is now almost 1 in a million (1 in 913,000). By comparison, your risk of dying in a motor vehicle accident is around 1 in 10,000. Pre-donating blood may be a safer option, but it increases your chances of having a blood transfusion—either of your own blood or someone else's—because you may become anemic before surgery.

organ meats, turkey and chicken (dark meat), dried fruits, whole grain cereals, peas, beans and dark green, leafy vegetables (e.g., spinach).

Jehovah's Witnesses

If you are a Jehovah's Witness, it is important to let your doctor know so he or she can discuss blood conservation strategies that do not involve transfusion. It is also important to find out what specific type of blood conservation program is available at the hospital where you are having surgery, because it can vary from hospital to hospital. For example, many hospitals offer closed systems to continuously recycle your blood, but others do not. Synthetic erythropoietins (e.g., Eprex, Aranesp) are not made from human blood, and your doctor may consider using one to boost your hemoglobin prior to surgery.

What Happens Next?

Once your questions have been answered, you've had the necessary tests and have signed the consent form, you're ready for the next and most important step—the surgical procedure. Chapter 7 tells you what will happen on the day of your operation.

Chapter 7

the day of your surgery

What Happens in This Chapter
- What to pack
- Hospital admission
- Surgical prep
- In the operating room
- Tips for friends and family

Knowing what is going to happen on the day of your surgery can prevent a lot of anxiety and inconvenience later on. Once you're admitted to the hospital, you will be assigned a bed and a nurse to look after you. Your medical team will do everything possible to help you relax and settle in. There may be a lot of waiting around before your surgery, but when you're in the operating room, things will move along quickly.

What to Pack

The hospital is a busy place and the staff there won't be able to provide you with many of the necessities you'll need during your stay. It's important to bring:

- A bag with basic toiletries (hairbrush, shampoo, soap, razor, shaving cream, toothpaste and toothbrush), a dressing gown and slippers ○
- A pair of roomy sweatpants with a flexible waistband for when you're discharged ○
- Assistive devices, such as a cane, braces, splints or prostheses ○
- Dentures, glasses and hearing aids ○
- Magazines, crossword puzzles or a good book to pass the time. You may be able to rent a television once you arrive at the hospital ○
- This book! ○

What you leave at home is as important as what you bring to the hospital. Unfortunately, there have been situations in every hospital where items have been misplaced, lost or even stolen.

Don't bring:

- Money and credit cards
- Your watch or other jewelry
- Work (your time in the hospital should be reserved for resting and healing)

Gearing Up for Surgery

Most hospitals will admit you on the day of surgery about 2 hours before the scheduled operating time. Either your doctor's office or staff at the pre-admission clinic should have informed you about when and where to show up. You may have already visited this part of the hospital and oriented yourself to it during your pre-admission visit.

Once you've arrived at the hospital, a nurse or caregiver will get you prepared for surgery. If you haven't already signed a consent form (page 106), you'll need to do so before your operation. There may also be some other final paperwork. You'll be asked to remove dentures, hearing aids, glasses and contact lenses. You may be asked to shower with a special antiseptic scrub before changing into a hospital gown. An identification band will be placed around your wrist; if you have allergies, you will get an additional colour-coded band. If medically indicated, you may also be asked to wear **antiembolic stockings** to decrease the risk of developing blood clots in your legs. You should have already undergone bowel prep (see page 108). The hospital staff will probably take care of shaving or clipping the hair in the area where your surgery will be. Most hospitals recommend that you do not shave yourself, as this may increase your chance of getting an infection.

Either in the ward or in the surgical holding area, a nurse or an anesthesiologist will start an **intravenous (IV) drip** of fluids and antibiotics in your forearm. You may be given an injection of heparin to thin your blood and reduce the risk of blood clots.

In the Operating Room (OR)

Next, you'll be taken to the operating room waiting area, usually referred to as the Surgical Admission Unit. This is a busy place full of hospital staff, as well as other patients awaiting surgery. In most hospitals, people walk from the holding area into the operating room with an escort.

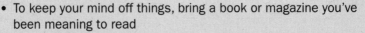

- To keep your mind off things, bring a book or magazine you've been meaning to read
- Ask any questions you have *before* you go into the operating room
- Give the following items to your companion for safekeeping: contact lenses, jewelry, eyeglasses, hearing aids, dentures and other prostheses

The operating room will likely feel cold. Your first impressions will be of very bright lights and a dizzying array of machines and instruments. The surgical staff will all be wearing scrubs, hats and masks, and will be attending to different tasks. You'll lie down on a narrow operating table in the centre of the room, where you will be strapped in to make sure you don't accidentally move out of place during the surgery.

"You get out of this waiting room bed and you walk to your surgery. And I thought, that is the worst experience they could ever give a guy. And when I talk to guys they say, 'You know what? You're right. That happened to me—I thought I was abnormal,' and I say, 'You're not abnormal; every guy has to do it.'"

JIM

Deep Vein Thrombosis

The complete immobility brought on by anesthesia in radical prostatectomy increases the risk of blood clots forming in the veins of the calf muscles. Under normal conditions, physical activity helps pump blood from the veins in the limbs back to the heart and lungs so that the red cells can be replenished with oxygen. Without the usual flushing action of movement, protein strands begin to collect along the inner walls of veins, trapping red blood cells and forming a clot, or **thrombus**. This jam of protein fibres and blood cells can grow in size until it partially or completely clogs a vein (**thrombosis**).

Since three main veins drain the calf, thrombosis in one of them won't make too much of a difference. The usual symptom of this kind of partial blockage is calf pain when standing or walking that is typically relieved by rest and elevating the leg. Sometimes, excess fluid seeps from small blood vessels into the surrounding calf tissues, causing a swelling called **edema**. Because it is difficult to detect, staff in the recovery room and nursing ward routinely monitor for any sign of **deep vein thrombosis** (**DVT**). If the clot loosens and begins to circulate (called an **embolus**), it can become lodged in the main arteries of the lungs—a life-threatening medical emergency. Symptoms of a blood clot do not usually appear until you are at home. If you notice pain, redness or swelling in the back of your calf or inner thigh, we recommend that you go to the nearest emergency department.

Although the risk of thrombosis is small (less than 1 in 100 in radical prostatectomy patients), you will likely be given anti-clotting drugs prior to the operation. Depending on your health history and risk factors, you may be given antiembolic stockings or pneumatic compression stockings that increase venous pressure and blood flow.

A blood-pressure cuff, as well as other monitoring devices, will be attached to your arm. An oxygen mask may be placed over your nose and mouth.

Radical prostatectomy using an open, laparoscopic or robotic approach takes about 2 to 3 hours. Whichever method of surgery, you will almost always be put into a deep sleep with a general anesthetic, and you won't remember the operation.

Friends and Family

Depending on your hospital's policy, friends and family members may be allowed to stay with you in the Surgical Admission Unit. Their presence often helps to relieve anxiety, and they can provide you with support when you're giving your consent or asking questions. Friends and family will not be allowed to stay with you after your transfer to the operating room. There is usually a waiting area for them if they wish to stay in the hospital during your operation.

> ! **[KEY POINT]**
>
> **If your friends and family** do not want to stay in the waiting area, they should leave details of how they can they be reached in the event that a member of the surgical team wishes to speak with them during your surgery. Most surgeons also like to talk to family or friends after the operation to let them know how your surgery went.

What Happens Next?

Next comes the main event—the actual surgery—although you won't remember much. But in case you're curious about what happens during your operation, the next chapter gives you a detailed account of your procedure.

Chapter 8

the surgical procedure

What Happens in This Chapter
- The anesthesiologist's role
- Step-by-step guide to radical prostatectomy

The big moment has arrived. Your surgical team will do their best to fix the problem and start you on the road to feeling better.

The Anesthesiologist's Role

Radical prostatectomies are almost always performed while the patient is under general anesthetic. The anesthesiologist may not be the same one you met at the pre-admission clinic, but he or she will consult your medical charts and history on the day of the surgery.

For a general anesthetic, an oxygen mask is placed firmly over your nose. You'll be asked to breathe slowly and deeply for several minutes to ensure that you get maximum levels of oxygen in your bloodstream. The anesthesiologist will then inject drugs through your intravenous line that induce sleep. At first, you may experience some burning through your arm veins or a metallic taste in your mouth—these sensations are normal. Once you are completely asleep, a breathing tube is inserted into your windpipe.

Some techniques will also involve inserting a spinal anesthetic. This is done by introducing a needle into the middle of your lower back and injecting a freezing agent into your spinal column. The spinal anesthetic helps control pain during and after the operation and reduces the amount of **narcotics** (pain medication) needed.

The anesthesiologist will use a number of devices to make sure your vital signs remain normal: a blood pressure cuff on your arm, 4 ECG electrodes to measure heart rhythm and an oximeter that analyzes your blood oxygen levels by gently squeezing one of your fingers. (See Figure 8–1 for a photograph of an operating room.)

Your Surgery

Depending on your surgeon's preference, once you're asleep you will be placed on your back in one of three positions: the lithotomy position, with your feet in stirrups; an open-leg position, where your surgeon just spreads your legs apart; or the standard straight-leg position. All work equally well. Antiseptic cleaning solution will then be applied over your belly and down to your penis and scrotum. A sterile drape is set up around the surgical field, and an **electrocautery grounding pad** is placed on your thigh.

For open surgery, an incision is made down your middle, from below your belly button to your pubic bone, although there are variations to this route of entry. A retractor is then placed in the incision to keep it open. For laparoscopic and robotic surgery, there are 4 to 5 port sites, or entry points. The incision is located near the belly button and is about 2.5 cm (1 inch) long.

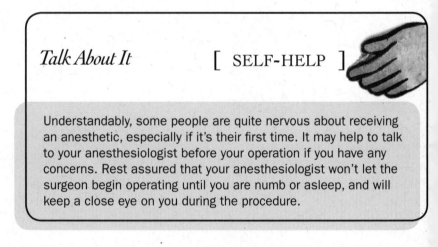

Talk About It [SELF-HELP]

Understandably, some people are quite nervous about receiving an anesthetic, especially if it's their first time. It may help to talk to your anesthesiologist before your operation if you have any concerns. Rest assured that your anesthesiologist won't let the surgeon begin operating until you are numb or asleep, and will keep a close eye on you during the procedure.

Figure 8-1 The Operating Room

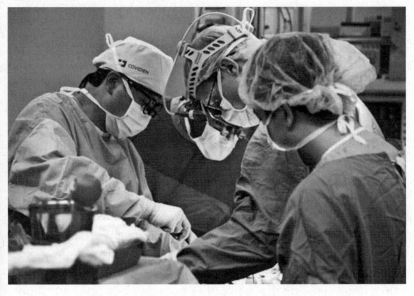

This is where you will have your prostate surgery

There are 6 basic steps to a radical prostatectomy
(see Figure 8–2):

1. The prostate is exposed and the connective tissue that holds
   it in place is cut away.

2. The **dorsal venous complex**, important blood vessels that
   sit directly on top of the prostate, must be tied off and cut
   to prevent bleeding.

3. Along the sides of the prostate run the nerves that control
   penile erection. During a nerve-sparing technique, these
   nerves are identified and separated from the prostate.

However, if a non-nerve-sparing procedure is being done, the nerves are removed with the prostate.

4. An incision is made to divide the urethra where it joins the prostate.

5. The prostate and seminal vesicles are dissected off the bladder.

6. The bladder is reattached with sutures to the urethra where the prostate once was.

When the bladder is reattached to the urethra, a catheter is put in place to bridge the new junction and will remain there for 1 to 2 weeks. Another plastic tube, called a **Jackson–Pratt drain**, may be inserted; it is then anchored over the bladder–urethra junction. The drain tube lies outside your body through a separate small incision beside the main one and is secured with a suture. The tube drains into an egg-shaped collector. This special collector continually sucks away any urine that might leak from the surgical join and cause infection. If urine doesn't leak (as is most often the case), the drain is usually removed within 1 to 2 days after the operation. Some surgeons do not use the drain since the chance of urine leakage is very low.

Figure 8-2 Radical Prostatectomy

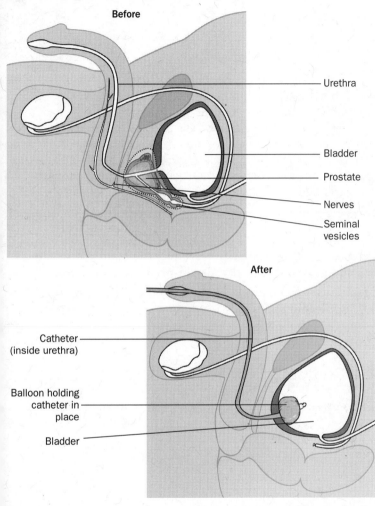

Before

Urethra

Bladder

Prostate

Nerves

Seminal vesicles

After

Catheter (inside urethra)

Balloon holding catheter in place

Bladder

This procedure involves removing the entire prostate and the seminal vesicles. Afterward, the urethra is rejoined to the bladder and a catheter is inserted into the urethra to allow urine drainage. The erection nerves may also be removed, although nerve-sparing techniques are the standard procedure unless they are not possible because of the extent of the cancer.

125

If you are offered a laparoscopic or robotic radical prostatectomy, learn more about these procedures on pages 90–91. They do the same thing as a conventional prostatectomy—they remove the prostate—but the surgery takes place through 4 to 5 small incisions in the lower abdomen, guided by a fibre-optic camera. Robotics allow 3D, high-definition vision with up to 10× magnification, giving surgeons a better view.

Depending on your surgeon's preference, the main incision is closed with either metal **staples** or **sutures** that dissolve on their own. A temporary dressing is applied over the incision, and you're transferred to the post-anesthetic care unit (PACU).

What Happens Next?

You'll wake up in the PACU and then be returned to the ward. Now your healing can begin.

Chapter 9

what happens after your surgery?

What Happens in This Chapter
- What to expect when you wake up
- Your catheter and other tubes
- Pain management
- Activities on the ward
- Going home

The first 24 hours after surgery are usually the toughest, but your medical team will make sure that your pain is under control and you're as comfortable as possible. You'll do lots of things to help your recovery along, such as breathing and coughing exercises, and taking short walks. Once you're able to eat and drink normally, and your surgical team feels that you are strong enough, you will be discharged home.

The Immediate Aftermath

Immediately after your surgery, you'll be transferred to the post-anesthesia recovery unit, or PACU. Although this clinical limbo can be a rather overwhelming place full of the strange sounds of monitoring equipment, hospital staff and reawakening surgery patients, most people don't remember much of their PACU experience. Waking up from anesthesia takes 1 to 2 hours, during which you'll experience moments of semi-consciousness followed by periods of deep sleep.

> "I remember waking up in a daze. I felt okay, but I was in a daze. I didn't experience any pain. I don't recall any pain at any time, but there was some discomfort."
>
> JIM

Return to the Ward

You'll feel groggy when you arrive back at your room. A nurse or caregiver will bathe you and take your vital signs (pulse, blood pressure, oxygen) to ensure that you're recovering as you should. You'll be given pain medication, made comfortable and instructed how to use the call bell should you need something.

Friends and Family [MORE DETAIL]

Usually family members and visitors aren't allowed in the PACU. Typically, they may have to wait 1 to 2 hours before seeing you. However, your surgeon or a member of the surgery team will contact your family once the operation is over to let them know how everything went. Once your caregivers feel your vital signs are stable, you'll be transferred back to the nursing ward to complete your hospital recovery.

If you feel nauseous or itchy, or experience a bladder spasm, let your nurse know so that he or she can make you feel better. Also, you'll likely feel thirsty and have a dry mouth, which can be relieved by applying a little glycerine or ice chips to your lips and rinsing your mouth. However, you won't be allowed to actually drink any water for about 6 to 12 hours, until your bowels have started to return to normal.

> "I remember my wife's words when I woke up: 'You're going to be fine. I talked to the doctor. You're going to be just dandy; he's got all the cancer out of you.' And that really set me feeling good."
>
> JIM

Your Catheter

After a radical prostatectomy, you will have a **Foley catheter** coming out of your penis. This was inserted into your bladder through your urethra during the operation. The Foley catheter, named after its inventor, Dr E.B. Foley, is a flexible tube, about 45 cm (18 inches) long, made of latex or silicone (see Figure 9–1). It is often coated with hydrogel to make both its internal and external surfaces completely smooth.

The diameter of the catheter depends on the nature of the urine being drained. Usually, a medium-sized catheter is chosen for prostate surgery, so there's enough room for tissue debris and blood clots to pass through it. A small balloon is attached to the end of the tube inserted into your bladder and is then filled with approximately 15 to 20 mL (0.5 oz) of sterile water. The balloon helps keep the catheter in place at the bladder neck. The exposed catheter tip is attached via tubes to the plastic urine bag by your bed. Special valves on the tube and bag allow them to be drained into a disposable container. Your surgeon may also use adhesive tape to place tension on the catheter; this will help stop the bleeding if required.

After a radical prostatectomy, you will keep your catheter from 7 to 14 days and leave the hospital with the catheter in place.

The drainage from the catheter may appear quite bloody at first and range from clear to dark burgundy. Don't be alarmed—this is normal. It takes only a few drops of blood to discolour a bag of urine. You may see that there are clots in the urine bag or a clot that passes along the side of the catheter—these are also normal and nothing to worry about. If you notice that your urine

Figure 9-1 A Foley Catheter

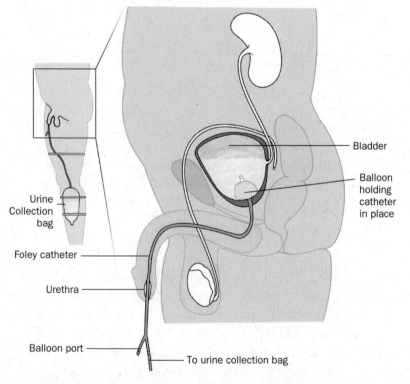

For a while after your surgery, you will pass urine through a Foley catheter, a long, thin tube held in your bladder by means of a small balloon. The urine drains into a bag that hangs by your bed. Once you are mobile, the bag can be strapped to your leg, underneath your pants.

is darker than normal, it's a good idea to increase your intake of fluids to help clear the urine.

Other Tubes

You'll slowly become aware of the other tubes and equipment that are still attached to you. You may have an oxygen mask or nasal prongs on your face to help you breathe. You will still have the intravenous line that was inserted into your arm before your surgery. Through your line, your medical team will give you pain medication, possibly

In the Ward...
It's All About You   **[MORE DETAIL]**

Here's a quick summary of how all those tubes and other equipment are speeding your recovery.

What is it?	What does it do?
Oxygen mask or nasal prongs	Helps you breathe
Intravenous line (from your arm)	Gives you pain medication, antibiotics and fluids
Foley catheter (from your penis)	Allows urine, blood and debris to drain from your bladder
Central line (an intravenous line in your neck)	An extra intravenous line (not always used)
Jackson–Pratt drain tube	Drains fluid from site of surgery (not always used)

antibiotics, and fluids until you begin eating and drinking normally.

You may also have another line, a **central line** (**CL**), in your neck. Your anesthesiologist used the CL to monitor blood pressure during your surgery. If your CL is not removed at the end of your operation, it will be shortly afterward.

Another tube that you may have after your surgery is the Jackson–Pratt drain in your abdomen. This drain tube is used to siphon away fluids that can accumulate around the surgical site.

Post-operative Pain

The key to getting through the pain after your surgery is, first, to understand what's causing it and, second, to tell someone if you feel that your pain isn't under control. While some discomfort is to be expected after your operation, the pain should not be unbearable. If you are in too much pain, you may find it difficult to get up and walk or do your breathing exercises, so don't try to be brave or tough it out.

With a general anesthetic, you may notice afterward that your throat is sore from the tube that was used to help you breathe during the operation.

You'll also gradually become aware of discomfort from your incisions and your bladder. Bladder discomfort, which is caused by your bladder muscles going into spasm, will feel like a strong urge to pee or a cramp-like sensation. Bladder spasms vary in intensity. Some men say they feel the spasm but it isn't painful; others say it feels like getting a charley horse in the calf. If you have bladder spasms in the hospital, unfortunately this means you may have

132

them the entire time the catheter is in place. In this case you may be prescribed medication to control them—**anticholinergics** such as oxybutynin (Ditropan) or tolterodine (Detrol). If you are free from spasms in the hospital you will probably stay free of them when you go home. Occasionally men say that they get a spasm when they have a bowel movement. This is normal and does not usually require medication. Keeping your bowel movements soft and being careful not to strain will decrease the possibility of spasms when having a bowel movement.

Pain Relief Medications

For pain relief you may be offered narcotics such as morphine and codeine, but increasingly a non-narcotic such as ketorolac (Toradol) is used instead. All these drugs can be given via your IV line, as tablets or as a suppository. Many centres are also using an anesthetic technique called **transversus abdominal plane (TAP)** block in combination with local freezing to the site of surgery and other medications. The idea of the TAP block is to cause a "road block" in the sensory nerve that normally allows you to feel pain in your abdomen, so that you hopefully need

less pain medication. As mentioned previously, anticholinergic tablets such as oxybutynin (Ditropan) and tolterodine (Detrol) can also be helpful for bladder spasms.

Less frequently, patients are offered **patient-controlled analgesia (PCA)** (see below).

> **!** **[KEY POINT]**
>
> **Some patients worry** about taking narcotics such as morphine and codeine because they are afraid that they will become addicted to them. However, it is rare to become dependent on narcotics when you are using them to control pain in the hospital because you are not given them for long enough.

If you experience side effects from these drugs, don't hesitate to mention them to your nurse. For more on medication side effects, see Chapter 16.

Pain Control at the Touch of a Button

After your surgery you may be offered a patient-controlled analgesia pump that is filled with pain medication and connected directly to your intravenous line. The pain medication is usually a narcotic. By pressing a button on this pump, you can give yourself an amount of medication specified by your doctor.

The PCA pump has a safety timer called a **lockout**, so you won't overdose yourself. If you press the pump button during the lockout time, you won't receive medicine because there is a limit to the amount of pain medication you can have. Once you press the button, the pain medicine should take 5 to 10 minutes to work.

Here is a list of do's and don'ts for your PCA pump:

DO
  • Press the button when you start to feel pain
DO NOT
  • Wait until your pain is bad before using the pump
  • Let others press the button on your pump
  • Use the PCA for gas pain or bladder spasms
  • Press the button when you are comfortable and sleepy

Get Busy Healing

Although a stay in the hospital may sound boring, you'll actually be kept quite busy working hard to help your recovery. One important task will be to breathe deeply and cough, up to 10 times every hour. These exercises expand your lungs and decrease the chance of fluid building up and the risk of pneumonia. Breathing and coughing post-surgery are particularly important if you're a smoker or have other lung problems, such as asthma. It's normal for coughing to be uncomfortable, especially if you have abdominal incisions, so try holding a pillow to your abdomen to absorb some of the strain.

You'll also be asked to wiggle your toes, pump each foot up and down (as if you were using your car brakes), and bend and straighten your legs. These exercises improve your blood circulation and reduce the risk of blood clots.

The next step is to start walking. It's important to get up and moving because it improves your circulation and reduces the risk of deep vein thrombosis (see page 117). Depending on the time of your surgery and when you return to the nursing ward, you'll be taken for a short walk that evening or the next morning. The first time on your feet is the most difficult, but your nurse will help you get going. You'll probably feel dizzy and quickly fatigued. Slowly, as you get more and more rest, you'll begin to feel stronger and walking will become easy again. Another sign that you're returning to normal is your ability to pass gas.

Going Home

When you're discharged, your nurse will give you a set of instructions to follow for your recovery at home. You will be discharged with the catheter still in place, so it's a good idea to have your companion with you on the day of your discharge. He or she can drive you home (and write down the nurse's instructions for you).

What Happens Next?

Once you're at home, it will be a time for you to rest and heal. You'll need to learn to care for your surgical wound and catheter, and there will be at least one follow-up visit to the urologist. You'll also have to keep an eye out for complications or side effects from your surgery.

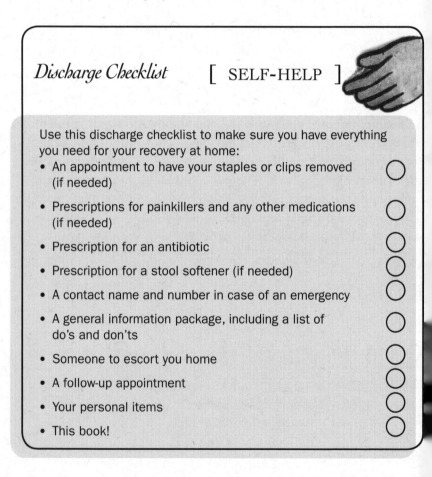

Discharge Checklist [SELF-HELP]

Use this discharge checklist to make sure you have everything you need for your recovery at home:

- An appointment to have your staples or clips removed (if needed) ◯

- Prescriptions for painkillers and any other medications (if needed) ◯

- Prescription for an antibiotic ◯

- Prescription for a stool softener (if needed) ◯

- A contact name and number in case of an emergency ◯

- A general information package, including a list of do's and don'ts ◯

- Someone to escort you home ◯

- A follow-up appointment ◯

- Your personal items ◯

- This book! ◯

Chapter 10

recovering at home

What Happens in This Chapter
- Caring for a surgical incision
- Managing your catheter
- Exercise, driving, flying, work, sex
- Follow-up with your doctor
- Side effects of radical prostatectomy

The surgeon's job is over, but now it's your turn to take the lead. You'll be responsible for caring for your incision and following up with your physician. Even though you'll have to exercise as part of your recovery, you'll still need plenty of rest and should return to your normal routine gradually. Most men experience urinary problems and sexual difficulties, at least temporarily, after a prostate procedure. There are several avenues open to you to deal with these common side effects of surgery.

Controlling Infection After Radical Prostatectomy

Human beings normally harbour vast numbers of bacteria on their skin, in their stomach, and in moist openings such as their mouth, nose, anus and urethra. Most are harmless and in some cases are essential for life itself. What's more, these less harmful bacteria take up space that might otherwise be colonized by more dangerous germs. Proper hygiene and a healthy immune system usually keep this microscopic "wild kingdom" in balance.

While infection of a surgical wound after prostate removal is rare, it may happen. It's slightly more of a challenge to keep your catheter infection-free for up to 2 weeks. Careful and diligent personal hygiene is a must to avoid the miseries of bladder and urinary tract infections. So, before you leave the hospital, your nurse will give you a crash course on how to look after your incision and catheter.

Surgical Wound Care

If you're nervous about having to care for your incision, don't be. It's no different than caring for a regular cut. The key is to keep the wounded area as clean as possible. Since incision sites are often left open to the air during your recovery period, frequent hand washing is the best way to avoid infection through contact. You can also feel free to shower regularly, even while your sutures or staples are still in place. On the off chance your wound does become infected, you'll be prescribed antibiotics.

Your incision will have been closed with either dissolvable sutures or surgical staples. Your sutures, which are under the skin and invisible, will be harmlessly absorbed by your body during the healing process and don't require a follow-up appointment. If the light plastic tape that covers your sutures falls off in the shower, it doesn't have to be replaced. If your surgeon used surgical staples you will have them removed either by your family doctor or during a short visit to your surgeon's office.

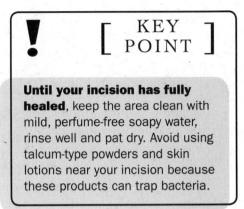

[KEY POINT]

Until your incision has fully healed, keep the area clean with mild, perfume-free soapy water, rinse well and pat dry. Avoid using talcum-type powders and skin lotions near your incision because these products can trap bacteria.

Catheter Care

While you were in the hospital, your nurse looked after your catheter. However, now it's your responsibility. Caring for your catheter is easy with a little practice and an understanding of how it works. You might want to review Figure 9–1 to familiarize yourself with the anatomy of your catheter (see page 130). A catheter uses gravity to drain urine from your bladder. So the first rule of living with a catheter is to always keep the drainage bag lower than your bladder. The bags come in two sizes. The smaller bag is for daytime activity and is attached securely to your upper thigh to reduce painful tugging on the catheter when you move. You can shower with the day bag in place, and it fits under track pants so that you can move around freely, which in turn promotes better drainage. The larger bag is for overnight use and lies by the side of your bed.

In the same way that running water stays fresh, urine usually remains sterile if it is routinely drained from your bladder. However, if urine sits around for a long time, it quickly becomes a breeding ground for bacteria that can infect your bladder and urethra. Keep an eye out for kinks in the tubing, as they can prevent your urine from flowing freely.

Another site that's vulnerable to infection is the urethral meatus, the opening where the catheter is inserted into your penis. Some urine normally bypasses the catheter when you sneeze, cough or have bowel movements, so strict hygiene is essential while you're living with your catheter. Gently cleanse the foreskin, the **glans**, the **meatus** and the catheter with antiseptic cleaning solution or soapy water at least twice daily. Pat dry. Make sure whatever you use to clean these areas is disposable—don't use the same cloth, wipe or towel more than once. Some doctors suggest applying a dab of antiseptic cream, such as Polysporin or Neosporin, to the meatus as an additional precaution against infection.

Also, make sure the foreskin isn't retracted behind the glans for a long period of time because this can restrict blood flow and cause your glans to swell painfully. Always wash your hands before and after cleaning the area around your catheter or your catheter equipment.

You should try to drink 2 to 3 litres (32 to 48 oz) of fluid a day to flush out your bladder. Water, tea and juice are best. Typically, your urine should be clear yellow, but it can fluctuate between a pinkish colour to a dark burgundy as old clots at the base of the bladder gradually dissolve. You may find that your urine becomes pinkish after too much activity, a bowel movement or an occasional bladder spasm, all of which can cause minor bleeding. Small clots may also pass down the catheter with bladder spasms and bowel movements, but this is nothing to be concerned about—"better out than in." Call your doctor if your catheter accidentally comes out—a rare occurrence.

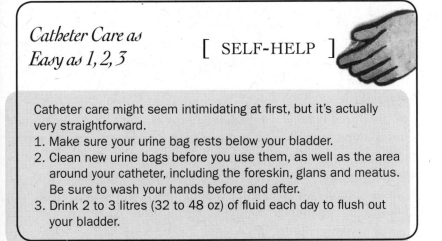

Catheter Care as Easy as 1, 2, 3

[SELF-HELP]

Catheter care might seem intimidating at first, but it's actually very straightforward.
1. Make sure your urine bag rests below your bladder.
2. Clean new urine bags before you use them, as well as the area around your catheter, including the foreskin, glans and meatus. Be sure to wash your hands before and after.
3. Drink 2 to 3 litres (32 to 48 oz) of fluid each day to flush out your bladder.

Maintaining Your Catheter Bags

You should wash out your used catheter bag each time you switch from the daytime bag (leg bag) to the nighttime bag (larger drainage bag). Liquid soap and water works well for this, or vinegar and water. Simply pour a small amount of liquid soap and water or vinegar into the bag, rinse with fresh water, shake well, and hang in the shower to drip-dry so it's ready for the next time. Urine should not be left in the bag, as bacteria will grow in it and act as a source of infection.

Return to Daily Activities

It's normal to tire easily after surgery, although the amount of fatigue varies from person to person. You're more likely to feel tired if you're older or not in good physical shape, so you may have to work a little harder to rebuild your stamina. It might help to eat frequent, small, high-fibre meals with plenty of fluids to make digestion easier and bowel movements less strenuous.

Exercise

For the first 3 weeks, exercise after a radical prostatectomy should be nothing more strenuous than walking. Start off with short walks and then progressively increase the distance as you gain your strength back. Rest when your body feels tired. Your recovery won't go faster if you push yourself too much. From about the fourth week after surgery, slowly return to your normal activities. Don't lift anything over 5 kg (10 lbs) for 6 weeks. You can go back to your sports activities after about 6 weeks, but increase your activity gradually and be guided by how well your body is tolerating the exercise. Swimming and baths should be avoided for 6 weeks, since soaking the incision may cause the top layers of skin to separate, leading to a larger scar. Bike riding should be avoided for 2 to 3 months—many men say the pressure of the bike seat may be very uncomfortable as it puts pressure on the perineum area where your prostate used to be. Contact sports such as hockey, football and soccer should be avoided for 2 to 3 months as well. For a detailed discussion of exercise, including tips and tricks to ease you back to fitness, see Chapter14.

Driving

After radical prostatectomy, you should avoid getting behind the wheel of a car for 2 to 3 weeks, to allow the lingering aftereffects of surgery and general anesthesia to resolve themselves. You should definitely not attempt to drive with a catheter in place as this will restrict your range of motion. It's worth bearing in mind, too, that in many provinces driving while "temporarily disabled" is an offence. Let someone be your chauffeur for a while!

Return to Work

After a radical prostatectomy, if you have a non-strenuous job with flexible hours, you should be able to get back after about 3 to 4 weeks, but keep in mind you may tire easily. If your work involves strenuous activity such as heavy lifting or straining, you will need at least 6 to 8 weeks.

Flying

Flying is possible within a few days after surgery, but bear in mind that you will have a catheter for the first couple of weeks, so you may wish to delay any trips until the catheter is out. Remember, too, that you should avoid lifting or straining for at least 6 weeks after surgery to avoid the risk of bleeding, so get help lifting and carrying heavy luggage. A heavy suitcase might also be your route to an incisional hernia, which happens when the increased internal pressure causes your internal organs to "pop" through the incision. This may happen regardless of the type of surgery, open, laparoscopic or robot-assisted laparoscopic prostatectomy.

Sex

After your surgery, feel free to start sexual activity whenever you are ready—ask your surgeon when you should start attempting it. Some men can achieve an erection shortly after the catheter is removed but feel too tired to do anything about it. Others find that nothing happens for an extended period of time. If your erection does not return, is not strong enough for penetration or does not last long enough, don't despair. As described in Chapter 13, there are lots of things you can do to regain your sex life.

Follow-up

"It took me 6 weeks off work, but I was pretty much back to normal after a month."

JIM

After radical prostatectomy, a key part of your first follow-up appointment is removal of your catheter. Your urologist may choose when to see you based on how quickly he or she thinks your bladder will heal. Or he or she may want to see you in order to perform a **cystogram** before removing your catheter, although most surgeons do not do this. If your surgeon does perform a cystogram, a contrast dye is injected through your catheter into your bladder until it is full. A type of X-ray image is taken, and then the dye is drained back through your catheter. If the dye leaks where the bladder and urethra have been reattached, then your catheter must remain until healing is complete. Either way, your "plumbing" will get a thorough check for leaks before you are sent on your way.

You'll need to stop taking any medication for bladder spasms one day before having your catheter out, because otherwise you might find it difficult to urinate (a condition called urinary retention). Catheter removal is usually simple. An empty syringe is attached to the catheter's balloon port (see Figure 9–1, page 130), and the balloon is deflated by sucking out the sterile water inside it. The catheter can then be gently removed. It is important to take deep breaths and relax your muscles so the catheter can slide out easily.

Possible Side Effects of Radical Prostatectomy (Open, Laparoscopic and Robotic Approaches)

Urinary Difficulties After Radical Prostatectomy

Excess scar tissue (urethral stricture) may build up in the urethra or bladder neck and cause trouble with urination for about 1 to 10 percent of prostatectomy patients. This problem is fixed by inserting a fibre-optic device called a cystoscope through the urethra, allowing the doctor to see inside via an eyepiece. A variety of special instruments for grasping, cutting and pushing aside scar tissue are then passed through extra channels in the cystoscope. Your physician will first try to crush the scarred area to dilate, or widen, the urethra and promote better urine flow. If this is unsuccessful, he or she will then cut away scar tissue during a procedure called a visual internal **urethrotomy**. Patients can be catheterized for a few days to a few weeks afterward.

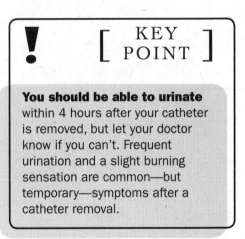

! [KEY POINT]

You should be able to urinate within 4 hours after your catheter is removed, but let your doctor know if you can't. Frequent urination and a slight burning sensation are common—but temporary—symptoms after a catheter removal.

Incontinence After Radical Prostatectomy

Virtually everyone leaks at first after a radical prostatectomy, to varying degrees. The good news is that the majority of men (90 percent) regain full bladder control in 6 to 12 weeks. About 1 to 10 percent of men have long-term mild incontinence, involving minor dribbling that may require absorbent pads, off and on. Less than 1 percent of men have such severe incontinence that a surgical solution such as an **artificial sphincter** is needed.

A common reason for incontinence is that part of the internal sphincter muscle or bladder neck was removed. During healing, the bladder may become irritated or experience a spasm, causing uncontrollable urges to urinate (urge incontinence). Abrupt pressure of mechanical stresses on the bladder, such as sneezing, coughing or laughing, can cause stress incontinence. Leakage can also be caused by an aging bladder that loses its muscle tone or a large belly pressing down on the bladder. It's also worth bearing in mind that when we get tired our muscles get weaker, so most men will find that dribbling increases in the evening as they start to get tired, but during the day and early afternoon they do not dribble as much. Alcohol or caffeine can also make the dribbling worse, so if you are dribbling more than you would expect you may want to cut back on these beverages for a while. Strenuous exercise may also increase the amount of dribbling.

Non-medical Treatment

For longer-term, mild leakage, a non-medicinal treatment option is **Kegel exercises**, which strengthen the pelvic floor muscles surrounding the urethra. Some studies show that Kegel exercises can cure the most common forms of incontinence after radical prostatectomy. You should notice an improvement in bladder control after 4 to 6 weeks. It's a good idea to start Kegel exercises before your surgery, so that they are already part of your routine when you return home. You can resume them once the catheter is removed after surgery. For detailed instructions on Kegel exercises, see page 209.

When you are tired, your muscles get weak and do not exercise as effectively. You should aim to perform your Kegels at a time when your muscles are at their strongest. For most men this is in the morning and afternoon.

> "When I came out of the hospital, what really aggravated me was the leakage, the incontinence. But I became conscious of going to the washroom regularly, and every time I passed one, I went—even if it was twice in an hour—and I retrained myself to stay dry."
>
> JIM

There is a wide array of disposable, absorbent pads and underwear that you can choose from to catch leaks. Finding a product that's effective and comfortable may take some trial and error. Believe it or not, you might want to consider disposable diapers for newborns. They are small enough to use as pads, very absorbent and cost much less than adult incontinence products. Bring an incontinence pad with you when you come to have your catheter removed, so you stay dry as you leave the appointment.

Recent advances in men's incontinence products have now led to a non-disposable option called STRIDE Everyday. With this product, the patented absorbent technology is sewn right into the underwear. The antimicrobial material fights odors, and the underwear is machine washable, so it can be reused.

Some incontinence products should be avoided altogether, such as condom catheters and urethral clamps. The condom catheter consists of a latex sheath that is placed over the penis. The urine collected by the sheath then empties through a tube into a drainage bag. Urethral clamps work by tightening a ring over the penis to close the urethra. If a condom catheter or clamp is too tight, blood flow can be constricted, causing painful swelling that's difficult to reverse. The clamps may also damage the urethra.

Medication

If your incontinence is persistent, there are some drugs your physician can prescribe to try and help you, although medications are rarely helpful with incontinence after radical prostatectomy. If your main problem is urge incontinence, a class of drug called anticholinergics may relieve cramps and spasms by relaxing the bladder's detrusor muscle. This group of medications includes the natural belladonna alkaloids (atropine, belladonna, hyoscyamine and scopolamine), oxybutynin (Ditropan) and tolterodine (Detrol). For more on incontinence medications, see Chapter 16.

Surgery

If your incontinence is particularly stubborn, a variety of surgical interventions can help. In some cases, microscopic collagen fibres can be injected into the muscles surrounding the urethra to add bulk to those tissues and make it easier for them to close. This procedure, however, is still at an experimental stage, and the long-term results are still unclear.

As a last resort, surgeons can implant an **artificial urinary sphincter**. This is necessary in less than 1 percent of patients with incontinence after surgery, but, when needed, it has a high success rate. The device consists of a silicone ring with an inflatable, fluid-filled cuff that is implanted around the urethra. It works when the urge to urinate activates a tiny pump in the scrotum that draws fluid from the sphincter cuff. The loss of fluid causes the cuff to shrink and lets urine pass down a small reservoir placed in the abdomen. After a few minutes, the pump automatically refills the cuff and re-blocks the urethra. This device can be extremely helpful, but mechanical problems are a possibility, such as unexpected deflation or partial filling of the cuff. If you do have an artificial urinary sphincter inserted, it is very important that you wear an alert bracelet (MedicAlert or similar) so that medical personnel are aware of it in the event of an emergency.

Erectile Dysfunction After Radical Prostatectomy

Avoiding permanent damage to your natural erections after surgery hinges on whether your surgeon can work around the nerve pathways that control the blood vessels in the penis, or, if this is not possible, graft in new ones (see page 87 for more on nerve grafting).

However, even if your "erection" nerves were removed, it does not mean that your sex life is over. Chapter 13 will walk you through your options for sex after surgery.

Rectal and Uretal Injury

Surgery is never without risks. Very rarely during prostatectomy, the wall of the rectum may be opened slightly. This is usually due to excessive scar tissue that could form between the prostate and rectal wall after the prostate biopsy. In most cases, this isn't a serious complication, and a few extra sutures during your surgery fixes the problem. You'll probably take just a bit longer to heal after your operation.

Cutting the ureter (one of two tubes that drain urine from the kidneys into the bladder) is also very rare, but a possibility. To correct this problem, your surgeon will insert a flexible tube, called a **stent**, along the entire length of the ureter and then suture the ends of the cut ureter back together. The stent allows the ureter's tissues to heal by shielding them from urine and providing an internal, stabilizing support system.

What Happens Next?

You've come a long way and your physical healing is complete. However, you may still have to make lifestyle changes and face the challenge of dealing with lingering worries. Chapter 12 gives you an overview of how to make the long-term changes you need and tools to deal with some of the feelings you might be having. Chapter 13 provides advice on restoring your sex life, and Chapter 14 covers the miraculous power of exercise.

Chapter 11

has my surgery worked?

What Happens in This Chapter
- Measuring success after surgery for prostate cancer
- The role of PSA tests
- Do you need more cancer treatment?

After your radical prostatectomy, the pathologist's report should be able to tell you whether the surgery has removed all of your cancer. If cancer cells are still present, you may be offered further treatment such as radiation or hormones.

Measuring "Success" After Surgery

When deciding whether your radical prostatectomy has worked, it is important to consider two issues: cancer control and quality of life.

Cancer Control

In order to decide whether your radical prostatectomy has successfully treated your cancer, the pathology report is key. PSA tests also have a role after your surgery.

The Pathology Report

After your prostate is removed, it is sent to a laboratory where a physician called a pathologist examines your tumour and prostate tissue under the microscope and produces the pathology report. This examination can take a while (2 to 4 weeks) because the prostate specimen needs to be properly prepared with chemicals and then sliced into very thin pieces before it can be examined.

As discussed in Chapter 3, by looking at your prostate in this way, the pathologist can determine the exact grade of the cancer and whether it is confined within the prostate gland. If the cancer is projecting outside the confines of the prostate gland, it is more likely to have spread. If it is projecting to tissue just outside the prostate gland, the pathologist will determine whether the tumour has reached as far as the edge of the surgery (or **surgical margins**). If the margin is "positive," it may mean that tumour cells were left behind, although this is not always the case (see Figure 11–1).

The pathologist will also find out whether the cancer has invaded other structures by examining the seminal vesicles and the part of the prostate gland that joins with the bladder. If your pelvic lymph nodes were removed, he or she will also examine them for signs that the cancer has reached them.

Figure 11-1 What Does Your Pathology Mean?

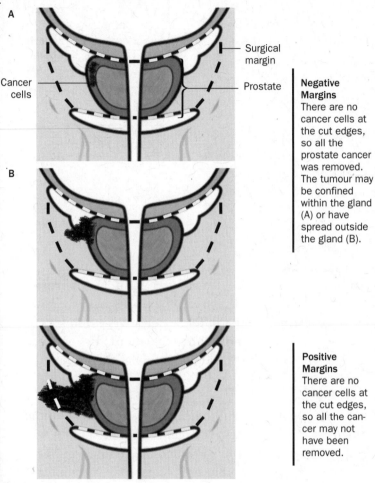

A

Cancer
cells

Surgical
margin

Prostate

B

Negative Margins
There are no cancer cells at the cut edges, so all the prostate cancer was removed. The tumour may be confined within the gland (A) or have spread outside the gland (B).

Positive Margins
There are no cancer cells at the cut edges, so all the cancer may not have been removed.

Once the prostate and surrounding tissues have been taken out, a pathologist will examine them to see if all the cancer was removed.

Once your oncologist has the pathology report, he or she will be able to tell you whether you need additional treatment for your prostate cancer and give you a reasonable prediction of your survival (**prognosis**).

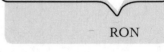

"I found out by reading the pathology report that cancer was found at the surgical margins. About 20 months' post-surgical, my PSA started to rise."

RON

You may have to wait a few weeks after your surgery for the pathology report, so try not to think about it until then. Focus on recovering from the operation!

Additional Treatments After Surgery

If your prostate cancer has spread outside the prostate gland, you may need some extra treatment such as hormonal medication or radiation in the area where the prostate was removed. If performed immediately after surgery, this extra cancer treatment is called **adjuvant treatment**. In some cases, treatment is given only if the cancer returns; this is called **salvage treatment**.

If the margins are positive or if the cancer has definitely spread outside the prostate, this extra treatment may take the form of radiotherapy. If your cancer has invaded the seminal vesicles or your pelvic lymph nodes, your oncologist may recommend hormonal treatments.

We know for a fact that such extra treatment works. Two large studies in the US and Europe found that patients who received additional treatment after surgery had better survival rates and chances of a cure than patients who did not get the additional treatment.

However, the most important question hinges around when should this additional treatment be given, that is, is adjuvant or salvage treatment better? The studies failed to discover which approach was better.

The advantage of doing adjuvant treatment is that it will treat any remaining cancer at its earliest point in development. The downside is that you may never actually have needed additional treatment at all. A study done at the Mayo Clinic looked at prostate cancer patients who had a positive margin after surgery, which would normally be considered a good reason to undergo adjuvant radiation treatment. Over time, only about 25 percent developed cancer recurrence—that is, 75 percent were cured by the surgery, and, if they had undergone radiation, it would have been unnecessary.

In other words, having a positive margin does not necessarily mean that the cancer was left behind. It could just mean that it reached the edges but did not extend beyond them. Sometimes a positive margin is expected if your cancer is so extensive that all three treatments are needed—surgery, followed by radiation and hormone therapy.

So the question of timing is still controversial, although many doctors now choose a wait-and-see approach—offering additional treatment only when there is evidence of cancer recurrence (i.e., salvage treatment).

The Role of PSA Tests
Even if the pathology report shows that your radical prostatectomy has removed all your cancer, your physician will want to keep an eye on you in case it returns. Regular PSA tests are the best way to do this. Because your prostate gland is the only organ that produces PSA, and your prostate has gone, all the PSA in your circulation should have gone too (see More Detail box).

What Does "Undetectable" PSA Mean?

[MORE DETAIL]

PSA levels in your blood will be undetectable after radical prostatectomy if all your cancer has gone. In practice, this may mean that your test results will say, for example, "less than 0.02 ng/mL," because this is the lowest limit that particular lab can detect. It can take up to 3 months for all the PSA to disappear from your body after surgery, so don't worry if your PSA is detectable over that time. If you are unclear what your PSA level means, don't leave your doctor's office until you are sure.

If your PSA never reaches undetectable limits after surgery or starts to go up, it means that there are still prostate cancer cells in your body producing PSA. The PSA could be coming from where your prostate used to be, or from other, tiny tumours that couldn't be detected before the operation (**micro-metastasis**). If this is the case, your oncologist will discuss with you whether to do nothing or whether you may need further treatments, such as radiotherapy or hormonal therapy.

It's important to remember that PSA measurements should be done on a regular basis for the rest of your life. Your oncologist will be able to tell you how often they are needed.

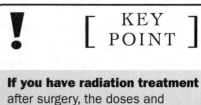

[KEY POINT]

If you have radiation treatment after surgery, the doses and duration of the radiation will be much lower than radiation that is given as primary treatment, and it is usually much more tolerable. It does not usually start until several months later, when you have recovered from your surgery.

Quality of Life

Quality of life is also an important consideration

after radical prostatectomy, when you are deciding whether the surgery "worked" or not. Apart from the natural concern about whether your cancer has gone, the two most important factors after surgery that will affect your quality of life are urinary control and sexual function.

> "Every year I go back for a PSA and my PSA registers as completely non-existent. But every time I go back I still have apprehension—what is it going to show?"
>
> SOL

When the catheter is first removed you will almost certainly leak urine and will need pads to protect your clothes. However, over the next few months your urinary control will gradually improve, especially if you do pelvic floor exercises regularly to build up your sphincter muscles. The majority of men have normal control of their urinary function by 3 to 6 months after surgery, although it may take as long as 2 years in a small minority.

If you continue to leak urine beyond this time and things show no sign of improving, you should discuss it with your oncologist, as there are several options that he or she can offer you (see pages 146–149).

With regard to sexual function, you will no longer be able to have erections if the nerves for erections were intentionally removed with the prostate gland during surgery. However, if one or both nerves were spared, or if a nerve graft was performed, then your erections can start to return as early as a few weeks after surgery, especially once your catheter is taken out. Bear in mind that erections, like urinary control, can take a long time to recover—as long as 2 to 4 years in some men. For more on erectile dysfunction and treatment options, see Chapter 13.

157

What Happens Next?

Life after radical prostatectomy can be a difficult adjustment at first, but be assured that over time most men find that their lives improve dramatically. Don't forget that your urologist, your oncologist and other members of your healthcare team are there to help, so don't hesitate to call on them. Remember, too, that you yourself are part of the team, so turn to Chapter 12 for ways you can help yourself make the most of your new lease on life.

Chapter 12

how you can help yourself

What Happens in this Chapter
- Understanding and dealing with emotions
- Managing stress
- Relaxation techniques
- Other lifestyle changes

Every man responds in his own way to the news of prostate cancer and the turmoil it brings to his life. Change is hard at the best of times, let alone when it comes in the form of a chronic or life-threatening condition. However, others have been there before you and there are lots of strategies for getting through this new phase of your life, such as finding support, learning to relax and improving your diet. There are also complementary therapies you might want to try. Every life change can be an occasion for personal growth and renewal, for sorting out priorities and reflecting on what you value most, and prostate cancer is no exception.

Managing Your Emotions

Many men present themselves as strong and stoic individuals. They tend to play down personal difficulties and setbacks to minimize the anxiety of those who rely on them. However, when you are coping with a serious illness such as prostate cancer, this show of strength may not be in your best interest. Understanding your own feelings and sharing your needs openly with others is not weakness—but the best way to tap into the strength of others around you.

Why Do I Feel This Way?

Most people like to be in control of their lives. Prostate cancer, or any chronic illness, can make you feel that you are no longer in control. You may have feelings of denial, anger, helplessness, powerlessness and confusion now that your future is more uncertain. In addition, you must cope with the fact that your illness is also causing emotional pain to those around you.

Communicate

Good communication is an important first step in managing your emotions. Communication allows you to alleviate your feelings by sharing them and to ask for help when you need it—both physical and psychological. Good communication also allows those around you to support you in the most appropriate way.

> "The more that I talked about it to different people, the more I found that people were giving me support, and that was giving me strength."
>
> JIM

Stay Positive

We know this is easier said than done, but try your hardest to keep a positive attitude. A positive outlook can have a major impact on your health. It will give you a feeling of control and decrease feelings of helplessness, reducing anxiety and stress. If you're having negative feelings, you might find it helpful to name them, either out loud or to yourself—"I am feeling anxious about my surgery"—before turning them to more positive channels—"but I can't do anything about my surgery now, so I may as well just enjoy dinner with my family tonight."

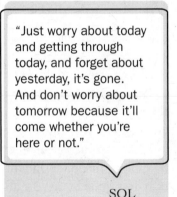

"In rock climbing, as in life, a small shift in attitude can solve an apparently insoluble problem."

MIKE LEASK, CLIMBER AND CANCER PATIENT

Live For the Present

We tend not to live in the present. Most of us live in the future, living our lives ahead of ourselves—hours, even days or weeks, ahead. We concentrate on what we have to accomplish, so thoughts of the future are generally associated with feelings of anxiety: "What happens if I don't get to work on time?" "What if something goes wrong with the surgery?" "What if I can't pay my bills?" The list is endless.

"Just worry about today and getting through today, and forget about yesterday, it's gone. And don't worry about tomorrow because it'll come whether you're here or not."

SOL

Many of us also live in the past. Continual reminiscing is associated with mourning or sadness because we are concentrating on what we have lost—our youth, our opportunities, our loved ones.

Living in the past or future uses up much of our precious time and emotional energy, and drains the pleasure from the present.

161

It is important to take possession of today and enjoy what we have here and now.

Support Groups

Prostate cancer survivors can provide excellent emotional support for those who are diagnosed with prostate cancer. They have been there and can understand the turmoil that you are

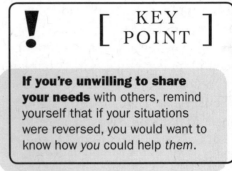

If you're unwilling to share your needs with others, remind yourself that if your situations were reversed, you would want to know how *you* could help *them*.

experiencing. It is comforting to know that you are not alone and that many have travelled the same road before you, and had to make the same difficult decisions you are faced with. Many men say it is reassuring to hear a prostate cancer survivor say, "I've been there." Many cancer centres and hospitals have prostate cancer survivor volunteers who have undergone special training to be a part of your healthcare team. They will support you throughout your journey, from diagnosis through to treatment and recovery. Support groups for spouses and partners are also available in many centres. Prostate Cancer Canada Network has a number of support groups across Canada for spouses and partners so they need not feel alone (see www.prostatecancer.ca).

Professional Help

Psychiatrists, psychologists and professionally trained counsellors can also provide emotional support and understanding, especially if you find that you cannot talk to family or friends. They will help you work through your personal or emotional issues in a confidential setting.

"Sometimes my wife said to me, 'well you don't need to tell everybody about it,' and I said, 'well, why not? I have nothing to be ashamed of.'"

SOL

Your physician's or surgeon's office will be able to refer you to professionals who specialize in cancer patients.

Religion and Spirituality

Let's not forget the mainstay of stressed human beings long before psychiatrists and support groups—religion and spirituality. More and more experts have begun to acknowledge the role of spirituality in emotional health and, by extension, overall health. A series of studies by researchers at Duke University recently determined that people who followed a religion tended to have stronger immune systems than non-followers and were less prone to depression and high blood pressure. They surmised that the faith of religious people gave them an enhanced sense of well-being and helped to reduce their levels of stress. Many men with prostate cancer find that their faith, as well as prayer, aids in relaxation and decreases stress; others say they find comfort by speaking with their priest, rabbi or other religious leader.

Managing Your Stress

Stress is a natural part of our lives—we cannot escape it. A serious illness such as prostate cancer is enormously stressful, but dealing with that stress may seem like the least of your worries right now. It is worth taking a look at practical ways to reduce your stress because this will help with your recovery.

In biological terms, stress is designed to help us cope with short-term demands (such as escaping that saber-toothed tiger), not long-term demands. Long-term stress is exhausting, affects our emotional health and wears down the immune system. This is not good for healthy people, and it is certainly not good for you. If you stay calm you will not only feel physically better; you will perceive things differently. You will be able to solve problems more effectively, view situations in context and balance options. These skills are especially important when dealing with illness.

Invest in yourself by taking the time to learn some stress-reduction techniques. They will not take away stress, but they will help you to react so that stress does not control your life.

In this section we briefly outline some ways to reduce your stress. There are also many self-help books and tapes available on this subject. Just check out the self-help section of your local bookstore or library, or "Resources" at the back of this book.

Sleep

Sleep-deprived people tend to become more easily angered and have less perspective on their emotions than people who are well rested with a regular sleeping pattern. Researchers have known for years that sleep and depression are closely intertwined. Getting a good night's sleep will refresh and revive both your body and mind, allowing you to think more clearly and restore some balance to your feelings. People vary in the amount of sleep they need. World leaders and insomniacs can survive with as few as 4 hours a night; other people may need as many as 9 or 10 hours. You will need to experiment to find your ideal level of shut-eye. Before your surgery you may have needed only a few hours' sleep, so you may be tempted to try and continue with your normal pattern. Be prepared to add more sleep after your surgery as a simple and safe way to restore your overall health.

Sleep Your Way to Good Health

[MORE DETAIL]

Getting regular, good-quality sleep can have a remarkable effect on your overall health—especially your emotional health.

Here are some basic "sleep hygiene" tips. Try one or more for a week and see if they make a difference.

- Avoid alcohol last thing at night
- Avoid all caffeine (cola, coffee, tea, etc.) after 5 pm
- Go to bed at the same time every night and do something quiet until you feel sleepy (e.g., listen to the radio, read)
- Avoid watching TV before you sleep—you could fall asleep over the remote and wake at 2 am feeling horrible
- If your partner snores or your home is noisy, wear ear plugs
- Turn off the phone ringer overnight
- Buy blackout curtains for your bedroom or try a temporary blackout with a dark towel or blanket
- Wear soft, comfortable pajamas or a night shirt (or nothing). Scratchy, restrictive clothing may be disturbing your sleep without your knowing it
- Is your bed comfortable? Say goodbye to those nylon sheets, toast crumbs and lumpy mattress!

If you're finding it hard to drop off or stay asleep, do a mental inventory of your sleep habits and environment. Simple changes can make a huge difference to the quality of your sleep. Take a look at the More Detail box above and try making one of these changes for just one week—you could be amazed by the results!

Realistic Expectations

A common source of stress is unrealistic expectations.
People often become upset about something, not because it is
intrinsically stressful but because it doesn't fall in line with what
they expected. If you set realistic expectations life will feel more
predictable and therefore more manageable. You will have an
increased feeling of control because you can plan ahead—and
your plans will pan out. For example, by reading this book after
your diagnosis of prostate cancer you are preparing yourself
psychologically and physically for what you can realistically
expect. Although we cannot take away what you have to go
through, we hope that this book will alleviate any unnecessary
stress by minimizing the surprises.

Humour

Humor is a wonderful stress reducer and a magical antidote to
many of life's upsets. Laughter relieves tension, both physically
and psychologically, and we often laugh hardest when we've
been feeling most tense. A good
laugh also provides perspective and
helps us feel closer to those who
laugh with us.

Relaxation Techniques

A good relaxation technique
gives your body a chance to rest.
By removing yourself from life's
demands and letting go for a while,
you will increase your feelings of
well-being and control, decrease
anxiety and panic, and help yourself
face each day's challenges calmly.
It may seem impossible to set aside
some time for relaxation—with

"I was joking with
people, saying they
got me with my shorts
down. Yeah, I was
embarrassed, but I was
happy to be alive. And
I was happy because
the people who were
teasing me, and that I
was teasing back, were
people that were on my
side, that had been very
supportive."

JIM

166

everything else you have to do! — but just one or two minutes a day is a good start.

Muscle Relaxation
When stressed, you tense your muscles, so learning to relax them, even under a lot of stress, is the most important first step. Relaxation tapes or CDs can help with this.

Start by sitting or lying somewhere comfortable and quiet, where you won't be disturbed. Close your eyes and focus on your breathing. Work toward slower, more regular breaths. Once you start to relax, concentrate on your head and imagine the tightness starting to ease. Continue to move down, repeating the process with your face muscles, neck, shoulders, and so on, all the way down to your toes. Feel yourself letting go; then continue to breathe regularly for a few more minutes.

Meditation
Meditation can be added to muscle relaxation. The goal is to quiet the mind but not empty it, so you may wish to think of meditation as a relaxation technique for the mind. At its most simple, meditation might involve repeating one positive word or phrase, your mantra, as you breathe in and out. As stressful thoughts intrude, they are acknowledged, then replaced by the word or phrase as you return to your mantra. Visualization (see below) is a more elaborate form of meditation.

Visualization
There have been many studies showing the power of the mind in medicine. If you doubt that there is a mind–body link, try recalling a frightening experience that you had. You will find that your heart is racing once more, and your palms are sweating. Imagine biting into a lemon — feel the saliva flow!

The goal of visualization is to harness the power of your imagination to help heal your body and encourage positive thoughts. This may be as simple as using images of lying on a beautiful warm beach to help you during relaxation, or imagining the colours of the rainbow, one by one, in time with your breathing. Or it could be more elaborate. One form of visualization, called **guided imagery**, can become quite involved; for example, you imagine your body undergoing surgery, then gradually healing. With **reminiscence therapy**, you focus on an event that gave you pleasure in the past and replay it in your mind.

Visualization is a powerful and increasingly popular technique, and there are many books, tapes and CDs available to help you explore it (see stress and relaxation in "Resources").

Sound Therapy
Listening to your favourite music can help clear your mind as well as being a good way to relax. CDs or downloads of relaxing sounds such as falling rain, the ocean or a bubbling brook also work well for many people.

Massage
Many people find a professional massage from a qualified massage therapist is a very good way to relieve stress, by physically relaxing strained or aching muscles.

"To get fully 100 percent, where you feel full of energy, it hasn't really happened yet. I still get days when I want to have a little nap in the afternoon."

RAY

Exercise and Weight

Exercise is good for everyone. It will increase your energy levels, help you sleep better, improve your cardiovascular system and may even boost your psychological well-being by increasing your self-esteem and relieving stress. For more on the miraculous powers of exercise, see Chapter 14.

Getting into shape is a good idea when preparing for surgery because it will help you recover faster. If you're not very athletic, get some guidance from your local YMCA, family doctor or a physiotherapist—or Chapter 14! It's never too late to start. Walking is an easy, inexpensive form of exercise.

Even if you are athletic, for the first 3 weeks after surgery walking is the only form of exercise that you should be doing. You'll probably be able to return to your normal exercise routine within 6 weeks after surgery, but build up gradually. It may take a few months to reach your pre-surgical stamina.

> **!** **[KEY POINT]**
>
> **After surgery, loss of muscle mass and tone** due to inactivity are serious concerns for older men who undergo prostate surgery. Even just 12 to 24 hours in bed can make you weaker. So any form of movement, even if it's shuffling around at home or taking short walks locally, is essential to maintain your strength during your recovery.

If you are overweight you may also wish to consider shedding a few pounds before surgery. For example, losing just 3 kilos (10 lbs) takes tremendous pressure off your hips, knees and feet, and reduces your risk of developing osteoarthritis. Getting rid of a large belly may also help relieve incontinence. We know this is easier said than done, but eating a well-balanced diet (see More Detail box) and getting more exercise may be all that's needed to reach a healthier weight.

Prostate Cancer and Diet

The University of Toronto Division of Urology recently conducted a review of scientific nutritional studies. They concluded that, although the scientific evidence is not always that strong, there does seem to be a link between some types of foods and prostate cancer. See Chapter 2 for more details on this.

Thinking of Using Complementary Therapies? [MORE DETAIL]

Complementary therapies are, generally speaking, not as widely researched as conventional drugs or surgeries, and the studies that do exist are often not up to the standard of conventional drug trials. This means that we don't always know about side effects or how people with different diseases might be affected, so be cautious. A therapy isn't safe just because it's "natural" (the natural world contains some of our most powerful poisons). There are, however, a surprising number of good studies, and the science of complementary therapies always makes for fascinating reading. For more on the link between diet and prostate disease, see Chapter 2.

What Is a Healthy Diet?

[MORE DETAIL]

Diets are hard, so let's keep the rules simple. Try to eat less food that is high in fat, especially saturated fat (all those hamburgers and hot dogs), and increase your intake of fibre (fruit, vegetables, whole grains). For help with this, follow the guidelines of a heart-healthy diet, which can be found in numerous websites or books. Visit the Heart and Stroke Foundation of Canada website (www.heartandstroke.ca) or Canada's Food Guide (http://www.hc-sc.gc.ca/fn-an/food-guide-aliment/index-eng.php) for healthy tips.

What Happens Next?

Surviving a serious illness such as prostate cancer is a remarkable accomplishment. With a little effort on your part, you can maintain and even improve your good health. Check out the resources at the back of this book for more information on staying healthy. You may also want to read Chapter 16 to learn more about the medicines your doctor has prescribed.

Chapter 13

sex after prostate cancer

What Happens in This Chapter
- What is sex?
- The basics of your reproductive anatomy
- Erections, orgasms and ejaculation: separate "systems"
- The effect of prostate cancer treatments on sex
- Erectile dysfunction: causes and treatment
- Working with your partner

The prostate gland is part of your sexual plumbing, so it's not surprising that all treatments for prostate cancer will affect your sex life to some degree. The disruption may be temporary, but it's something to be prepared for. Sex is a complex business and means different things to different people. Some men are comfortable with a scaled-down sex life; others want to regain what they had before. Either way, being prepared for what might happen, understanding why it happens and being aware of the many treatment options available will help you and your partner rediscover this important part of your lives.

Why Talk About Sex?

When a man hears he's got prostate cancer, sex is unlikely to be the first thing that springs to mind. The word "cancer" is associated with facing mortality, while sex is a private, intimate pleasure. However, once the first shock of the diagnosis has worn off, it is perfectly normal to start worrying about how the various prostate cancer treatments might affect your sex life. As discussed in Chapter 5, most of the treatments for prostate cancer will have some effect on your ability to obtain and maintain an erection—either permanently or temporarily.

Many people, especially older men, are uncomfortable talking about sex—even to their partners—and in some cultures it is actually taboo. Even fairly "open" men may hesitate to mention sex to their physician or nurse because they feel guilty for bringing up the subject when everyone else seems focused on saving their life: "you've got cancer—who cares about sex?" In fact, if your sex life is important to you, it does deserve plenty of consideration. Your healthcare providers are committed to helping you regain the best possible quality of life that you can have, and sex is part of that. Even if you have never discussed such private matters with anyone before, at least consider talking through your sexual concerns with your healthcare team. Remember, they work in a urology clinic: there is nothing they have not heard or seen when it comes to men's intimate lives.

Be warned that we use pretty graphic language in this chapter. We believe that, when it comes to sex, it's important to use clear, factual words that everyone can understand. However, an important message of this chapter is that sex is more than medical facts. By using the words of poets from across the centuries, we have tried to show that all men everywhere share the same hidden corners of human passion that no medical words can ever describe.

What Is Sex?

The answer to this question may seem pretty obvious. You may, quite reasonably, reply: "sex is sexual intercourse." Well, yes it is, but in this chapter we're going to broaden the definition a bit. Need convincing? Take a look at the poem below.

If sex is just sexual intercourse—if it's all just about hard penises and penetration—why does the man want to see his lover's face?

> She lowers her fragrant curtain
> wanting to speak her love.
>
> She hesitates, she frowns—
> the night is too soon over!
>
> Her lover is first to bed,
> warming the duck-down quilt.
>
> She lays aside her needle,
> drops her rich silk skirt,
>
> eager for his embrace.
> He asks one thing:
>
> that the lamp remain lit.
> He wants to see her face.
>
> **Chinese Poet Liu Yung**
> **AD 987–1053**

The reality is that sex is a complex, intricate, intensely private experience that is different for every person, every couple, every time. There is no perfect sex life, no right way to perform sex and no absolute measure of "success." There are couples who communicate well, are sexually creative and enjoy their intimacy. Other couples may have a regular sex life but do not really communicate well and have little intimacy. Then there are those who do not really communicate, are not intimate and are rarely (or never) sexually active. Only an individual and his partner can decide what sex means to them, and whether their sexual lives are satisfactory for both of them.

> "We've made a lot of discoveries on the sexual side since my surgery, a lot of discoveries. We've discovered there's a lot more to the whole thing than the sexual act, once you get away from the erection focus. You have to be willing to look for alternatives, explore new ways to make love. The key is to open and honest."
>
> MARK

It's worth remembering this if you experience sexual difficulties after your prostate cancer treatment. Even healthcare providers are often guilty of reducing the sexual experience to the ability to achieve an erection, the rigidity of the erection, how long the erection lasts, and so on. Sex is much more than an erection. In your previous life your sexual experience may have revolved around your erection and your ability to achieve one, but be assured that in your new life, you can get more creative than that—if you want to. Later in this chapter we will explore the possibilities.

The Machinery: The Male Reproductive Anatomy

Although sex isn't all about the anatomy, it is helpful to have a thorough understanding of how it all works. As always, knowledge is power.

The Brain

Although men tend to get rather focused on their penises, perhaps the most important sexual organ is the brain. You don't get to tell your brain what you find arousing: your brain tells you! Emotional excitement is an extremely important component of sexual enjoyment and intensifies a man's perception of any physical sensations of the penis. Conversely, the brain contains a man's attitudes and past experiences, which may help (or hinder) sexual enjoyment. Given that the brain has such a crucial role in sex, it is easy to understand why anxiety, fear, stress or depression may interfere with an erection.

! [KEY POINT]

There is no anatomical reason why your orgasm or your libido should be affected by prostate cancer surgery, radiotherapy or brachytherapy. This is because the nerves that control erections and the nerves that control sensations are completely different. The "sensation" nerves hug the side walls of the pelvis and are well away from the prostate. So even if your erection nerves are damaged and you cannot have an erection, you can have pleasurable sensations and achieve orgasm.

The Penis

The penis is one of the most versatile organs in the body, since it has several roles. Most obviously, it is the male external reproductive organ—the piece of machinery that allows a man to father children.

However, as a highly sensitive erotic zone, it has a separate role in providing pleasure and reinforcing a man's relationship with his partner. If you doubt that these roles are separate, consider this: if the penis were just about fathering children, why would men have sex when they aren't trying to conceive? It is useful to bear these two roles in mind when we are thinking about erectile dysfunction. In the normal course of events you *do* need an erection to father children. You do *not* necessarily need an erection to achieve pleasure or have a wonderful relationship.

The third important role of the penis is, of course, for urination.

! [KEY POINT]

Contrary to the belief that sex is for the young, a study by the University of Chicago published in the prestigious *New England Journal of Medicine* has shown that sex is lifelong for many men. Researchers found that 73 percent of men aged 57 to 64 years old are sexually active; 53 percent of 65- to 74-year-olds still have sex—and so do 26 percent of men aged 75 to 85.

This remarkable piece of engineering is made up of two parts: the shaft and the **glans penis**. The shaft is the main part of the penis and contains a network of tissue that can rapidly fill with blood. The glans penis is the cone-shaped end or head of the penis, which is where the **corpus spongiosum** ends. The small ridge that separates the glans penis from the shaft of the penis is called the **corona**. The **frenum**, or **frenulum**, is where the corona makes a little V shape, also known as the man's G spot. A narrow tube called the **urethra** runs the length of the penis, and both urine and sperm leave the body through this tube (see Figure 1–1 on page 4).

These structures each have their own sensations, and each contributes in its own way to a man's total sexual experience. For some men the frenum, or frenulum, is the most intensely sensitive part of their whole penis. For others it may be the glans. For uncircumcised men the foreskin is a very sensitive area.

The Perineum

A significant portion of the penis lies inside the body. It can be felt underneath the area of skin called the **perineum**, which is directly behind the base of the scrotum. This portion of the penis also responds to manual stimulation. The perineum is a highly sensitive erotic zone, considered by some men to be the most sensitive part of their body after the penis.

The Scrotum

The **scrotum** is the bag of skin lined with muscle that hangs below the penis and contains your testes or testicles. The testicles make sperm, and to do this they need to be cooler than the inside of the body. The muscles of the scrotum pull the testes closer to the body to protect and warm them in situations of extreme cold, for example when jumping into a cold pool. The scrotum is sensitive to touch for many men and is another important erotic zone.

The Testes (Testicles)

The **testes** are the two small organs found inside the scrotum. They make sperm and produce the male hormone testosterone. Testosterone is the key hormone that gives men their "maleness"—their strong muscles, deep voice and body hair. The testes are another erotic zone and are incredibly sensitive to touch.

Internal Reproductive Organs

The key reproductive organs that are not visible from the outside are the **epididymis**, the vas deferens, the seminal vesicles and of course the mighty prostate gland itself. The anatomy of these organs is described in detail on pages 5–6. Their roles in a man's sexual experience are described below.

The Epididymis

This small organ perches on top on the testicles, and its job is to store sperm until they are needed. When a man ejaculates, the sperm are moved from the epididymis into the vas deferens (see below). Most men are unaware of their epididymis; they can't usually feel it, and it doesn't have a direct role in the sexual experience.

Vas Deferens
These narrow tubes represent the first stage of a sperm's journey out of the body. They transport sperm out of the epididymis and into the urethra, via the seminal vesicles, for ejaculation. They are crucial for fatherhood but do not have a direct role in sex.

Seminal Vesicles
These tiny sac-like glands lie behind the bladder and release a fluid that forms part of semen. Like the vas deferens, they do not have a role in the sexual experience.

Prostate Gland
Last but not least is the prostate gland itself. As described elsewhere (see page 6), the prostate gland surrounds the neck of the bladder and its role is to secrete a slightly alkaline fluid that forms part of the seminal fluid, which carries sperm. It is sensitive to pressure and touch, so in the right context it can be an erotic zone. The prostate can be manually stimulated with a finger, by anal intercourse or by massage of the perineum. Unfortunately this will not be possible if your prostate is removed.

Erection, Ejaculation and Orgasm: Separate "Systems"

In healthy men **erection**, **ejaculation** and **orgasm** are one seamless experience, so it may come as a surprise to realize that they are, in fact, completely independent biological functions. This is good news because it means that if you lose one, you don't lose all. After prostate surgery you will no longer have ejaculate, but erections and orgasms are still potentially on the cards. Even if you can't manage an erection, you can still have orgasms. This section looks at how each of these processes works in healthy men.

Erections

Erections may be thought of as a simple hydraulic event in which blood vessels at the base of the penis relax, allowing blood to flow into the spongy tissue in the shaft of the penis. At the same time, the "exit" blood vessels squeeze shut. This leads to an increase in pressure in the penis and the development of rigidity (hardness).

> "I achieved an orgasm within a month although I wasn't getting an erection at all. You had to get used to that. What I didn't realize was that you'll still have sensation and orgasm, even if there's no erection. This was really important knowledge. The biggest surprise I had."
>
> MARK

The blood vessels at the base of the penis are controlled by nerve signals from the brain that pass into the penis through the erection nerves (see Figure 1–2 on page 6).

Erections can be triggered by direct stimulation of the genitalia or, thanks to the ingenuity of the brain, a wide variety of mental triggers. Fantasy or mental imagery can be as powerful at triggering an erection as a real sensory stimulus such as the scent of a familiar perfume or the sight of a lover.

Needless to say, at a minimum, erections need intact, functioning nerves and good blood flow to the penis. However, mood plays a part, too, because the brain is the gatekeeper of those all-important nerve signals. This is why, as mentioned earlier, anxiety and fear over erections can interfere with the erection process and, in effect, become a self-fulfilling prophecy.

Ejaculation

There are two stages to an ejaculation: the **emission phase** and the **expulsion phase**. During the emission phase, the first stage of ejaculation, the seminal fluid is gathered inside the prostate gland, where it is joined by newly minted sperm from the vas deferens to form semen. In the expulsion phase, the semen is expelled out of the penis by strong contractions of muscles at the root of the penis. This takes 3 to 10 seconds.

> "Leah did a great job of telling me what to expect—in graphic detail! She was very positive, chances were for a full recovery within a year, but she emphasized it could be a couple of months before anything happened. The part that was hard to understand was what it would be like to experience a 'female orgasm.' I just didn't know what to expect."
>
> ROB

Obviously, for ejaculation to happen, a functioning prostate gland is needed to produce semen, and the internal muscles must be strong enough to force the semen out of the penis.

Orgasm

The reflexive flood of pleasure and release known as an orgasm is a function of your brain, not your penis. This psychological event results from stimulation of your erotic zones, which are well-endowed with hundreds of sensation nerves. Strange as it may seem, you do not need an erection or a release of seminal fluid to achieve an orgasm; you just need a functioning brain. If you don't believe us, ask any woman.

Erectile Dysfunction After Prostate Cancer Treatments

Erectile dysfunction (ED) is defined as being regularly unable to achieve an erection or maintain it long enough for satisfying sexual relations.

As discussed earlier, a serviceable, natural erection needs three things:

- A good blood supply
- Healthy erection nerves
- A brain "willing" to become erotically stimulated

Problems in any of these areas can create erection difficulties, so ED can be caused by many types of traumas and illnesses, some permanent but many temporary.

All of the treatments for prostate cancer can potentially cause problems with erections. Prostate surgery can cause ED by removing or bruising the erection nerves or damaging the arteries. Radiation or brachytherapy can also damage the nerves and blood vessels. Hormone treatments for prostate cancer can cause erection problems by lowering blood levels of testosterone, which lowers libido.

Any disease that affects the arteries can cause erection problems, because the blood supply to the penis is affected. For this reason, men with diabetes, high blood pressure, high cholesterol, coronary artery disease

> **! [KEY POINT]**
>
> **The only thing a couple** may lose when prostate cancer strikes is natural penetration. Both partners can still feel desire, sexual pleasure, arousal, orgasm and satisfaction.

or previous strokes or heart attacks commonly have ED. In fact, this fact is so well-known to physicians that ED is now seen as an early warning of cardiovascular problems down the road. When a man's doctor asks about sexual prowess at the annual physical, he or she is not just being nosy!

Erection difficulties are often associated with disorders involving the nerves, such as spinal cord injuries, Parkinson's disease, multiple sclerosis or Alzheimer's disease—both because of nerve damage itself and the depression that often comes along with these serious conditions. Depression is commonly linked to ED, although untangling cause and effect can be tricky here: both depression and the treatments for depression can cause ED; conversely, ED can lead to depression. Hormone disorders such as thyroid disease and low testosterone levels can also affect erections, as can serious illnesses such as kidney or liver failure. Finally, sleep apnea, obesity and obstructive pulmonary disease can cause ED, although the reason for the link with these disorders is unclear. Again, depression or fatigue—or hidden cardiovascular problems—may be at fault.

Medications can also affect a man's ability to achieve and maintain erections. As we mentioned earlier, antidepressants are well-known culprits in this regard. ED is also a possible side effect of blood pressure pills, cold medications, hormone treatments and tranquilizers, among others. Excessive alcohol, smoking and narcotics such as heroin and cocaine can also cause erection problems.

Solutions for Erectile Dysfunction

Counselling
As we said at the beginning of the chapter, the brain is the most important sex organ of all. So, if you're having sexual difficulties after prostate cancer treatment, the logical starting point is the

mind—not the body. Treatments that focus on the erection itself are described later in the chapter.

Professional counselling for anxiety-based erection difficulties resolves the problem about 50 to 70 percent of the time. Even if you are considering going right to a medical solution for ED, counsellors will be helpful in guiding you and your partner to agreement on a treatment choice. However, perhaps the most important role of a sexual counsellor is in helping the couple improve their sexual communication and lovemaking skills so that they can continue to have a satisfying sex life even if there are no erections, or make "better" use of the erections that the man does have.

The major advantage of a counsellor is that he or she is not your lover. He or she is an external source of strength and insight for both of you, who is not involved emotionally with the situation. Counselling may simply take the form of coaching and education— providing practical advice on new lovemaking techniques as you adapt to changes in your body, or new ways to connect that are not based on sexual activity.

Counsellors can also open the lines of communication between you and your partner. Evidence shows that the partner plays a key supportive role in treatment and therapy. Sexual dysfunction is a shared sexual problem that can have detrimental effects on men and on their partners if a proactive approach is not maintained by both. Your partner may have concerns and needs that you are not aware of, and a counselling session provides a non-emotional setting in which to discuss them. You also have concerns and needs. Most men do not want to be pitied or viewed as a cancer victim, but as a cancer survivor. However, many men feel isolated because they are afraid their partner will reject them due to their change in sexual capacity. Counselling provides a safe forum in which to air these thoughts and feelings.

Learning to Reconnect
It is not uncommon for couples to stagnate in their sexual routine. Creativity takes too much time and energy, and couples often take the relationship for granted. The diagnosis of prostate cancer is a wake-up call for many couples, who find that they have new appreciation for each other after their brush with mortality. However, the association of penetration and sexual intimacy is so strong for many people that they give up on their sex lives after cancer treatment, asking themselves, "why start what you can't finish?" But, as we said earlier, sexual intimacy is not all about a hard penis and penetration. Erectile medications enhance erections, but they do not create desire. Reconnecting as a couple plays a much larger role in a satisfying sex life than taking medications or using mechanical aids.

In our experience, many couples find that the diagnosis of prostate cancer has rekindled their sexual connection because it has made them explore new ideas for expressing physical and emotional intimacy. Relearning how to connect can be half the fun! Many couples say that trying new techniques and exploring each other's body can be a very erotic experience. Some find that, even if a new technique did not produce the expected results, they had a great time trying. Humour and patience are key, and it's important not to get too hung up on things that "don't work." Allow yourselves to laugh, and try something different the next time.

Maximizing Enjoyment (for You)
Many men say that after prostate cancer treatments, learning how to lengthen the arousal period, while delaying orgasm, is an important part of maximizing enjoyment from sex. Like any exercise, practice makes perfect.

When the penis is flaccid, touch will seem little different from touch on any other part of the anatomy, which can be discouraging. However, as arousal begins, the nerve endings concentrated in the penis start to become more sensitive and reactive to the touch. The first sexual feelings may be rather unfocused, but as arousal proceeds, sensation will increasingly seem to emanate from the groin area. The longer this stage can be maintained, the more powerful and enjoyable the orgasm will be. Many men believe these sexual sensations occur only in the penis, but many other places in the groin area are quite sensitive as well. Learning to fully enjoy these sensations and psychological urges for a longer period of time without moving directly on to orgasm is something that some men must learn. But the results are well worth the effort, both in terms of your own enjoyment and in the fulfillment of your sexual partner.

Sex After Prostate Cancer [SELF-HELP]

- We keep saying this, but we'll say it again: sex is more than a hard penis and penetration
- You still have all your erotic zones, and you can still achieve orgasm
- Learning to reconnect is half the fun!
- Don't be afraid to try new techniques
- Talk candidly with each other
- Don't assume you know what your partner wants—ask
- Be patient
- Have fun
- Don't give up
- If you're finding it's all getting too tense, consider a sexual counselor
- Counsellors will give you practical lovemaking advice as well as provide a safe forum for discussing intimate matters

Maximizing Enjoyment (for Her)

It often comes as a surprise to men to learn that many women don't consider a hard penis to be the centre of their sexual world. This is good news, not bad news. Your concerns that you won't be able to "satisfy" her if you can't penetrate may be misplaced. Generally speaking (and there are no hard and fast rules here), there are three important things that researchers have discovered about women when it comes to sex:

> Without [the drug] I don't get much of an erection although I sometimes achieve enough for penetration. My wife is very helpful and encouraging. You just have to work harder at it, be open about it, take a bit longer, work on different techniques and experiment around a bit.
>
> MARK

- The context of the sexual experience is very important. Unlike most men, who can become aroused quickly by mechanical stimulation, the mechanics are only one component of women's enjoyment. Feeling a connection to her partner, feeling needed and desired, are crucial to a woman's sexual enjoyment. "Foreplay starts at breakfast" is the key thought here.
- Women need more sexual stimulation than men to reach orgasm. This is good news for you as you try to lengthen your own period of enjoyment. If you are working together to arouse each other, your partner may not be as impatient as you imagine.
- Vaginas aren't very sensitive. The most erotic zone in the woman's body is the clitoris. This is not so surprising, since the clitoris is the equivalent of the male penis. It is very rare for a woman to achieve orgasm by penetration alone (although not unknown). If you have not paid much attention to her clitoris before, now may be as good a time as any.

Despite your own fears and worries, try and understand your partner's concerns. She may be just as worried about her sexual needs as you are, but feels guilty raising the issue when, after all, you have just survived a life-threatening illness. On the other hand, some post-menopausal women consider sex long since over and done with and are rather dismayed at the prospect of renewing sexual relations after their partner's surgery. As with all aspects of your lives together, communication is the key.

Maximizing Enjoyment (for Male Partners)

If your sexual partner is a man you may also need to adjust your normal sexual routine. Explore new variations of foreplay and communicate with your partner to see what does and doesn't work for him. As we advised for female partners, try to understand your lover's concerns about his own sexual needs and communicate openly about the new situation. For in-depth help with your needs as a gay man, see Chapter 15.

> "I can't get erections, I can't penetrate. But I've been married for over 30 years. I've got a great marriage. And I always say creativity.... If a man's got a tongue and ten fingers he can be very creative and have sex.... I still have orgasms, but I have dry orgasms. So my sex life right now is satisfactory."
>
> JIM

Medical Treatments for Erectile Dysfunction

Men who experience permanent erectile dysfunction after prostate cancer treatments have several options for regaining firm erections. These options include oral medications (tablets), penile injections or suppositories, vacuum devices and penile prostheses. Sexual aids vary greatly in effectiveness and invasiveness (i.e., how easy the treatment is), with the most invasive forms generally being the most effective.

The erections that you had before your prostate cancer treatment are a good guide to the erections that you can expect with

> *Doing, a filthy pleasure is, and short;*
> *And done, we straight repent us of the sport:*
>
> *Let us not rush blindly on unto it;*
> *Like lustful beasts that only know to do it:*
>
> *For lust will languish, and that heat decay.*
> *But thus, thus, keeping endless holiday,*
>
> *Let us together closely lie and kiss,*
> *There is no labour, nor no shame in this;*
>
> *This hath pleased, doth please, and long will*
> *please; never*
> *Can this decay, but is beginning ever.*

Petronius Arbiter, Roman poet
(1st century AD)

medical intervention after your treatment. If you had erection difficulties before your prostate surgery, don't expect better erections after surgery just because you're now taking tablets.

If you are considering some medical assistance for your erections, talk to your healthcare team before doing anything. Never buy devices or tablets (e.g., Viagra) from the Internet or borrow from a friend. You risk serious injury to yourself and your penis.

PDE5 Inhibitors

The treatment of erectile dysfunction was revolutionized in 1998 by the launch of sildenafil (known to millions as Viagra) — the

189

first oral treatment for ED. Viagra was the first of a group of drugs called the **phosphodiesterase-5 (PDE5) inhibitors**, which now include Cialis (tadalafil), Levitra (vardenafil) and Staxyn (vardenafil orally disintegrating tablet, which is a "melt-in-your-mouth" version of Levitra).

PDE5 is an enzyme concentrated in the penile erectile tissue, which turns off an erection. Medications such as Cialis, Levitra, Staxyn and Viagra relax the smooth muscles in the penis by blocking this enzyme, allowing blood to flow into the penis and making the penis harder.

PDE5 inhibitors were a breakthrough because they do not create an erection—a sexual stimulus is needed. This means that you can take a tablet in anticipation of sex, but if the moment is not right no erection occurs, unlike with the prostaglandins, which almost always create an erection—appropriate or not (see pages 178–180).

The PDE5 inhibitors seem to work equally well in men across the board. They all seem to work to some degree after nerve-sparing prostate surgery, too, although it's difficult to compare the drugs directly because all the studies use different measures of success. One of the ways to assess how well an ED drug works is to ask the men "Did you successfully complete intercourse?" Using this measure, Levitra was successful in 60 percent of men 1 year after surgery and Cialis was successful in 41 percent of men

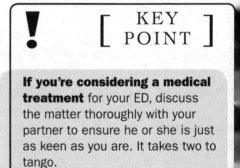

[KEY POINT]

If you're considering a medical treatment for your ED, discuss the matter thoroughly with your partner to ensure he or she is just as keen as you are. It takes two to tango.

3 months after surgery. Viagra "improved" the erections of 43 percent of radical prostatectomy patients.

It is important to note that one or both erection nerves must be present for these medications to work. Levitra, Staxyn and Viagra need to be taken within 4 hours of anticipated sexual activity. In general, Cialis can be taken up to 36 hours prior to sexual activity, thus providing a longer window of opportunity for sexual spontaneity. Unfortunately, after most prostate cancer treatments, you may find that this 36-hour window is reduced to about 6 hours.

Side effects of the PDE5 inhibitors are generally mild and include headaches, a bluish tinge to the vision, flushing and nasal congestion. Tylenol can be taken for the headache, and a nasal spray can help alleviate nasal congestion. Antihistamine tablets should not be taken with PDE5 inhibitors as they will counteract the effects of the PDE5 inhibitors.

If you have cardiovascular disease, are taking nitrate medication and are thinking of using the PDE5 inhibitors, you must talk to your physician first. Cialis, Levitra, Staxyn and Viagra *must not be used by men who are taking any form of nitrate medication on a regular basis*. Whether taking nitrates in pill, spray, paste or patch form, the combination may have dangerous effects on blood pressure. If you use nitrate medications only occasionally, your cardiologist or urologist may consider that a PDE5 inhibitor is an option. Always take your specialists' advice on these matters.

It is important to note that anxiety may alter the effectiveness of PDE5 medication. Before starting this medication it is important to discuss with your partner what you will do if it doesn't work as well as anticipated.

Use It or Lose It

Until recently, many physicians believed that erectile dysfunction after nerve-sparing prostate surgery could be staved off by giving their patients a nightly dose of a PDE5 inhibitor for several weeks following surgery. This so called **sexual rehabilitation** seemed logical, based on theories of why ED happens, small studies involving just a few men, or studies that measured things like nightly erections.

However, arguably the most relevant test of any ED drug is—can a man successfully complete intercourse? A recent large, well-conducted study by the manufacturers of Levitra showed PDE5 inhibitors make no difference to a man's ability to complete sex when used as daily prevention (although they still work well when taken as needed).

This study also showed something else interesting. Men who were on the placebo had surprisingly low rates of ED, compared with results from previous studies. Why was this? The researchers concluded that a form of "sexual rehabilitation" had been going on, after all. All the men in the year-long study had been told to regularly "attempt sex," either by masturbation or with a partner. By regularly increasing blood flow to the penis, even if they didn't get a full erection, the men had been keeping their erectile tissue healthy and reducing the risks of permanent ED down the road. When it comes to erections, it's obviously "use it or lose it"!

Prostaglandin Therapy

A therapy for erectile dysfunction that is popular among some men is alprostadil, a type of **prostaglandin**, which is a powerful promoter of blood flow. This therapy induces an erection within 5 to 20 minutes, and it lasts for up to an hour.

There are two routes for taking alprostadil: an injection directly into the spongy part of the penis (e.g., Caverject) or a tiny suppository that is inserted into the urethra (MUSE). Many men start with MUSE as it is less invasive than the needle. Both therapies are described next.

> "I'm now getting partial erections and the doctor said to keep trying: if you're seeing progress, there's still hope you'll get back what you had before. Even if it seems there's not much there, you have to work hard at it, even if you don't get instant satisfaction."
>
> MARK

Penile Injections

Several medications can stimulate erections if you inject them directly into the side of your penis with a needle. Although most men would rather do almost anything than inject their penis, in fact these medications are not particularly painful. Caverject is an injection of prostaglandin E1, described above. A product called Regitine is a combination of papaverine and phentolamine. "Triple mix" is a combination of all three of these drugs.

Penile injections relax the smooth muscles within the penis, promoting blood flow. When combined with stimulation (foreplay), penile injections usually produce a firm erection. Success rates are reportedly around 85 percent.

The downside of injections after prolonged use is that the penis may develop scarring, which can cause it to be permanently curved. There is also a small risk of a prolonged, inappropriate erection (**priapism**) requiring medical intervention. If your erection lasts longer than 4 hours after a penile injection, you need to seek medical attention as you may suffer tissue damage to the penis. About one-third of men have a dull ache in the penis following an injection, but this usually fades after a few minutes. In rare cases, penile injections can cause a sudden drop in blood pressure, resulting in fainting.

Urethral Suppository

MUSE is a tiny tablet (micro suppository) of prostaglandin E1 that is inserted in the urethra via a special applicator. This medication works in a similar way to penile injections but avoids the use of a needle. MUSE works best if inserted into the urethra after urination. After insertion, the suppository is massaged into the urethra through manual stimulation of the penis. Standing may increase blood flow to the penis after inserting MUSE. The reported success rate with MUSE is 57 percent.

Vacuum Constrictive Devices (VCD)

A VCD is a pump that a man places over his flaccid penis when he wants to have an erection. There are several different versions available: some are pumped by hand, while others use a battery. VCDs are most commonly used for erection problems that have an identified medical cause.

With a VCD, the air is pumped out of the cylinder, creating a vacuum that draws blood into the shaft of the penis, causing the penis to swell and become erect. The erection is maintained by placing a **constriction ring** over the base of the penis before the pump is removed. Success rates are reported in the 85 to 92 percent range.

One of the downsides of a VCD is that part of the penis that is inside the body will not fill with blood, so the penis will only be erect beyond the placement of the ring, causing the penis to pivot. The pivoting does not interfere with intercourse. Another downside is that the penis may become cool to the touch, especially if the ring is left on too long, which some partners don't like.

As with other medical therapies, a vacuum device should only be used with direction from a physician, and there are some important safety measures to follow. The ring should not be left on for longer than 30 minutes since it is, in effect, cutting off the blood to the penile tissue. Since the device can also cause bruising of the penis, a VCD should not be used by men who are taking blood thinners such as Coumadin, Fragmin or ASA (Aspirin).

Penile Prosthesis

A penile prosthesis (**penile implant**) is usually considered the treatment of last resort. Implants are reserved for men who suffer from erectile dysfunction with an identified medical cause and who have failed previous ED aids or treatments, or are unwilling to try less radical sexual aids.

Penile implants can be inflatable or permanently semi-rigid and involve inserting the implant into the shaft of the penis. Inflatable implants are pumped up before sex by means of a fluid reservoir in the abdomen and a pump-and-release valve tucked into the scrotum, then deflated after sex. With semi-rigid implants, as the name implies, the penis is neither fully rigid nor flaccid, and thus is more difficult to conceal under clothing. Semi-rigid implants also permanently place pressure on the interior of the penis, and this may cause tissue damage.

The downside of all implants is that they involve major surgery, and, despite the risks and inconvenience, may not work that well. Cost is also a factor. Overall, long-term satisfaction with penile implants is around 85 percent.

Medical Treatments for Erectile Dysfunction

Treatment	Advantages	Disadvantages
PDE5 inhibitors (Cialis, Levitra, Staxyn, Viagra)	• Success rates for full intercourse 40–60% • Minimally invasive (easy to take) • Maintain spontaneity	• May not work • Cost • Can't be taken with nitrate medications • Won't work if erection nerves removed
Penile injections	• Success rates up to 85% • Can work even if erection nerves removed/damaged • Useful if can't take PDE5 inhibitors	• Penis discomfort • May not work • Cost • Risk of prolonged, inappropriate erection • Scar tissue in 10–15%, which can curve penis • Fainting (rare)
MUSE	• 57% success rate • No needle • Can work even if erection nerves removed/damaged • Useful if can't take PDE5 inhibitors	• Penis discomfort • May not work • Cost
Vacuum constrictive devices	• Success rates 85–92% • Do not require medication or surgery	• Cost • Can cause bruising • Can't be left on longer than 30 minutes • Can't use with blood thinners • Penis may be cool to the touch so not a natural feel
Penile prosthesis	• 85% satisfaction rates reported • One-time surgery • Avoids risk of curved penis caused by penile injections • More relaxed foreplay with no change in skin sensation	• Infection in approximately 2% of men, requiring removal of the prosthesis • 15% of implants fail, and surgery is required to repair/remove prosthesis; may be embarrassing with a new partner

Ejaculation After Prostate Cancer Treatments

After most prostate cancer treatments, men will notice a decrease or absence of ejaculate. Radiation therapy and brachytherapy both decrease the amount of ejaculate, and after prostate surgery there will be no ejaculate at all, as the prostate and seminal vesicles are removed at time of surgery.

Orgasm and Libido After Prostate Cancer Treatment

Many men believe that if they can't have an erection, they can't have an orgasm. Hopefully you will be convinced by now that there is no anatomical reason why your orgasm or your libido should be affected by prostate cancer surgery, radiation or brachytherapy.

Orgasms

When we talk to men after surgery, we hear the full range of comments. Some men say their orgasms are about the same; a small percentage say the orgasm is still pleasurable but slightly less intense; others say that their orgasm is even better than before treatment. How is this possible? According to the men themselves, the greater emphasis on foreplay after surgery or treatment, combined with rediscovering the erotic zones of their bodies, has resulted in orgasms that are much more intense. These men have learned to channel their sexual energy into the sensations and the orgasmic experience, instead of focusing on their erection.

As discussed earlier in the chapter, the sensory nerves that control skin sensation and orgasm are different to the nerves that control the blood flow to the penis. These nerves hug the pelvic side walls and are well away from the prostate surgical area. The feeling in the genital area does not decrease, and sensations are not affected. Men should experience exactly the same sensation during orgasm, down to the rhythmic pumping of the muscles at the base of the penis, as they did before surgery.

There is one caveat, however. If your prostate is an erotic zone for you, your sexual experience may be altered if your prostate gland is removed. For men who have radiation and brachytherapy treatments, which do not destroy all the prostate tissue, the prostate may remain an erotic zone.

"I assumed, incorrectly, in order for a man to experience an orgasm it required full ejaculation—I never understood before that they are separate and distinct mechanisms. At first I found the orgasm less intense, which was alarming. I called Leah right away and she said this was due to surgical trauma and would resolve in time. She was right—it did."

ROB

Libido

After prostate surgery, radiation or brachytherapy, there is no anatomical reason why a man's desire for sex should change. Your sexual drives, desires and libido are not directly affected by these treatments. However, the anxiety associated with the diagnosis of prostate cancer and the challenge to achieve an erection can interfere with the libido. Prostate cancer frequently disrupts a couple's relations in ways that can affect quality of life for both the patient and his partner.

A diagnosis of prostate cancer often precipitates concerns about mortality, disability and a changing self-image. For many men, a change in their sexual functioning causes loss of identity that can be more devastating than the loss of ability to engage in intercourse. Sexual function, potency and physical appearance are intimately involved in the concept of self-esteem and can play as great a role as the physical disease itself in the impact of cancer.

Thus, the psychological impact of sexual dysfunction may be just as devastating and life-altering as the actual diagnosis and treatment of the cancer. Studies show that 60 percent of men report "moderate to severe" distress related to sexual dysfunction. In one study looking at men 1 year after surgery, 12 percent said they were afraid the cancer would return and 40 percent reported concerns about sexual dysfunction.

The reaction of partners may also contribute to this emotional turmoil. In the studies, men reported that, once the fear of cancer recurrence subsided, the single most distressing after-effect of prostate cancer surgery was accepting and adapting to sexual dysfunction and its impact on interpersonal relationships. Remember, too, that depression—and antidepressant drugs—can blunt sexual desire; depression is common after a major illness such as prostate cancer.

Needless to say, all these factors can profoundly affect libido and reduce a man's interest in the bedroom—the place where all his fears and anxieties seem to come together.

If this is the case for you, consider talking to a counsellor and getting some of these fears out into the open. Sharing your concerns with someone who is not emotionally connected with the situation may be all that is needed. If you are on an antidepressant that seems to be dampening your sexual desire, your physician may switch you to a medication that has fewer sexual side effects.

Although most prostate cancer treatments do not directly affect libido, there is one exception. Hormone treatments for prostate cancer reduce levels of testosterone and decrease libido in about 80 percent of men, making it difficult to be sexually aroused and to orgasm. The remaining 20 percent of men may retain their interest in sex but need much more genital stimulation to achieve orgasm.

Sad to say, there are no magic potions to increase libido. If there were a true aphrodisiac out there, every urologist and urology nurse would have bought the stocks long ago.

Single Men

As if a diagnosis of prostate cancer was not stress enough, single men often experience quite distinctive stresses to those of their married colleagues.

Not only do single men lack the emotional and physical support of a partner, but many fear that the diagnosis of cancer—and the side effects of cancer such as erectile dysfunction—may lead to rejection and they will die lonely. Self-esteem, body image and masculinity are important for all men, but doubly important to single men who are seeking new relationships, whether just for a good time or for a more substantial long-term relationship. Although able to achieve successful erections with medical aids or devices, many men are reluctant to disclose information about their prostate cancer, as they still consider this taboo or are fearful of the response they may receive.

If you are in that position, consider this: most of us judge ourselves more harshly than others do. When deciding whether to disclose information, put yourself in the other person's shoes. How would you feel if the roles were reversed? Would you be put off an attractive person just because he or she was a cancer survivor? If the person is not interested because you are bravely battling the effects of cancer treatment, he or she is probably not worth your time anyway!

What Happens Next?

Most people's sex lives have changed throughout their lives and adapted to changing circumstances. If you now need to explore new ways of enjoying your sexual experience following prostate cancer treatment, be positive. It's just another interesting chapter in this most interesting of human experiences.

"What would I say to a man worried about sexual recovery? Just one word: patience. Give it time— things will continue to improve. Mother Nature's powers of healing are remarkable."

ROB

We know you care deeply about your patients and will do everything you can to get them through their prostate cancer. However, even healthcare professionals sometimes hesitate to raise the matter of sex—especially if the man doesn't raise it first. As healthcare providers we need to be able to openly discuss the issues that affect our patients' whole being, not just the parts that we deem important. We need to talk more frankly than ever before.

Come up with a plan in your clinic to assess, treat and support each patient who experiences sexual difficulties as a result of his cancer diagnosis. Ideally, start the assessment *before* treatment begins.

The goals of your assessment and counselling should be to:
- Increase the couple's awareness of the impact of prostate cancer on their intimate life
- Manage their expectations
- Determine the most effective ED treatment (if required)
- Maintain intimacy and sexual activity
- Help them adapt to changes in sexual activity
- Help them come to terms with the new situation

Chapter 14

exercise, the miraculous medicine

What Happens in This Chapter
- The benefits of exercise
- Your exercise plan

There are many benefits to exercising before, after and even during your prostate cancer therapy. Regular exercise can increase your strength and help you recover faster. It can also help you reduce your risk of developing other diseases, deal better with stress and improve your sex life. Even though it can seem hard to follow through with a fitness program, especially if you're not feeling well or not used to exercising regularly, there are small steps you can take to help you maintain a healthy activity level as you undergo treatment.

The Benefits of Exercise

Exercise is an important part of staying healthy. The good news is anyone can participate in an exercise program at any stage of life and benefit from it. Staying fit is especially important if you are undergoing treatment for prostate cancer, because it can help you heal faster and reduce treatment-related side effects.

How Exercise Can Improve Healing

If you are fit before your surgery, your recovery may be easier, faster and more successful. That's because exercise will strengthen tissues such as your heart and blood vessels. If you have stronger, healthier tissues, your wounds will heal better, including the blood vessels and nerves around your penis that need to work properly for you to have erections. There are also specific exercises that you can perform to minimize any urinary incontinence you might experience after surgery. Exercise is even an effective way to manage the fatigue and stress you are feeling as you go through your cancer treatment journey.

The Power of Exercise

[MORE DETAIL]

Staying fit can help to prevent disease and improve your quality of life. Exercising helps you:
- Reduce your risk of developing cardiovascular disease, high blood pressure, high cholesterol, stroke, type 2 diabetes and certain kinds of cancer
- Strengthen your immune system
- Maintain a healthy weight
- Develop healthy bones, muscles and joints
- Reduce fatigue
- Deal better with stress
- Improve your sex life
- Control incontinence
- Sleep better

Healthier Tissues

Being physically active will give you an advantage during your prostate cancer treatment because your tissues will be stronger and more likely to heal better. Exercising even a little bit causes your tissues to be flooded with oxygen and nutrients. Physical activity also improves your blood circulation and reduces your risk of developing conditions that affect your blood vessels, such as high blood pressure, type 2 diabetes and **atherosclerosis** (plaque that blocks the arteries). If your tissues are healthy and blood can circulate more easily throughout your body, you will not only have more energy and be able to perform physical tasks with less effort, but also be able to heal faster and more completely after surgery.

Studies on Exercise and Sex   [**MORE DETAIL**]

Studies show that men over 50 who exercise 3 to 5 hours a week have better erections and are 30 percent less likely to experience erectile dysfunction. Other research shows that if you exercise frequently, your "sexual age" will be years younger than your actual age. You may even find yourself more receptive to sex and experience greater sexual desire when you exercise regularly.

Better Sex

Boosting your healing potential through exercise has another major post-surgery advantage: better sex. The improved cardiovascular and general tissue health that comes with regular exercise lowers your risk of developing permanent erectile dysfunction as you recover from your treatment. Your healthier blood vessels, including the ones in your penis, will not only mend better following surgery, but also allow blood to flow through them more easily and produce stronger erections. Even in men without health problems, exercising regularly can lead to harder, longer-lasting erections. This is why in urology we often say "heart health is penis health."

"I knew surgery was coming and I also knew I was a little bit overweight. I thought if I lost that abdominal fat my [erection] nerves would be easier for the surgeon to see. I lost 25 pounds before surgery and felt fantastic. The night after the surgery the surgeon came in smiling like a Cheshire cat. My [erection] nerves were like neon signs, they were so easy to isolate. He said I had a great chance of maintaining erectile function."

SOL

Aside from better blood circulation to the penis, exercise can provide you with more strength and endurance during sex. You'll be able to experiment with different positions that require greater physical control as well as enjoy longer lovemaking sessions. Having the freedom to get creative in the bedroom can be particularly useful if you're challenged by erectile dysfunction. For more information on sex after prostate surgery, read Chapter 13.

Control Incontinence

A common side effect of prostate surgery is urinary incontinence, or the inability to control when you urinate. Although going to the gym or for a walk won't help reduce incontinence, a very specific form of pelvic floor exercises called Kegel exercises (see page 209) can help you strengthen the muscles that are responsible for urination before your surgery, so that it is easier for you to regain control of urinating after treatment.

More Energy

Exercise can also give you the strength to go about your daily tasks during and after your treatment. One way that exercise helps you do this is by reducing fatigue, which is a common side effect of cancer and cancer treatment that affects up to 95 percent of patients. A 2004 study published in the journal *Cancer* showed that prostate cancer patients who exercised during radiation therapy were less fatigued and physically stronger by the end of their treatment than patients who did not exercise.

In addition to causing fatigue, androgen deprivation therapy can lead to weight gain and bone and muscle mass loss, making it hard to perform daily activities such as climbing stairs. Preserving the tissues that are responsible for keeping you strong and reducing body fat through exercise will allow you to lead a more normal and energetic life as you recover.

Reduce Stress

Exercise is a great natural way to reduce your stress levels, which is especially important when you're dealing with the anxiety of facing a major illness such as prostate cancer. Exercising stimulates certain chemicals in the brain that leave you feeling happier and more relaxed. You will feel calmer immediately after a workout and will be better able to handle all kinds of life stresses if you exercise regularly. Plus your appearance will improve, which can give you more confidence in your daily activities, including during sex.

Your Exercise Plan

Getting and staying strong as you go through treatment and recovery is essential. The following section gives you tips on how to start an exercise program if you haven't exercised regularly before and addresses some of the concerns that men who are already physically fit often have when they are diagnosed with prostate cancer.

Getting Started

Whether you're new to exercise or have always been physically active, it is important to begin by setting goals. One of your goals may be to reduce fatigue. Or you may want to build your strength or flexibility. Maybe you really want to increase your endurance or lose 10 pounds. Writing a list of what you want to accomplish will help you come up with a realistic fitness plan and follow through with it. Just be sure to talk to your doctor before starting or modifying any exercise program. Your doctor can give you guidance on the kinds of exercises you should be doing, how often you should be doing them and their intensity.

How to Do Kegel (Pelvic Floor) Exercises [SELF-HELP]

1. First you have to find your pubococcygeal muscles. Do this by stopping your urine flow midstream—the muscles that are contracted while your urine is stopped are the pubococcygeal muscles that you tighten to perform Kegels.
2. Once you've identified which muscles are used during Kegels, you don't have to perform the exercises while urinating. Simply contract the pubococcygeal muscles for 7 to 10 seconds, as tight as you can. This should feel as though everything is being lifted in an upward motion. You should NOT be tightening your abdominal muscles.
3. Relax for 7 to 10 seconds and then repeat.
4. It is recommended that you do 45 to 60 repetitions of this exercise a day—try 30 in the morning and 30 in the afternoon.

Doing the exercise periodically throughout the day will help you build the number of repetitions you can do. It is important to try and work up to 30 to 45 repetitions at once. Many men say that when they start to perform Kegel exercises, they sometimes feel numbness or pain when increasing the number of repetitions. This is perfectly normal. Remember this takes practice, so don't get discouraged. We usually tell men it takes more than a week to build up the stamina to run a marathon; the same goes for building the pubococcygeal muscles. Start off slowly and keep practicing to build yourself up.

Kegel Exercises

One of the first exercises that you need to incorporate into your routine are Kegels (see Self-Help box). Practice Kegels before your surgery and afterward, once your catheter is removed.

A nice side benefit of Kegels is that they may also improve sexual function. When you get really experienced, you can perform Kegels just before orgasm to delay ejaculation; when you want to have your orgasm, fully relax all your pelvic floor muscles.

If You're New to Exercise

Beginning an exercise plan can seem intimidating if you are not used to working out. But even if you have not exercised regularly before, it's never too late to start. Keep in mind that your workouts do not have to be strenuous or extremely time-consuming to be effective. All you need to do is adjust a few habits and set aside a bit of time to make exercise a normal part of your life.

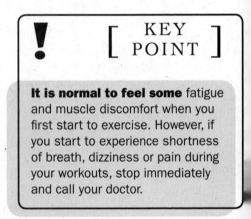

[KEY POINT]

It is normal to feel some fatigue and muscle discomfort when you first start to exercise. However, if you start to experience shortness of breath, dizziness or pain during your workouts, stop immediately and call your doctor.

Your workouts should eventually incorporate the two basic kinds of exercise: **aerobic** and **resistance**. Aerobic exercise improves your cardiopulmonary fitness (the strength of your heart and lungs). Examples of aerobic exercises include walking and cycling. Resistance training, such as lifting weights, will improve your muscle strength and endurance.

Choosing the Right Workout

If you're new to working out, your doctor will probably recommend adding some less intense exercises that are short in duration to your daily routine. It is important to start slowly and closely monitor how you feel during the new activities.

An easy way to figure out whether you're working out at a moderate intensity is to use the talk test. While you're exercising, you should be able to carry on a conversation. If you are having trouble speaking, you are exercising beyond a moderate intensity.

You don't have to buy fancy equipment or join a gym or sports league to start being more active. Try a few simple modifications to your daily routine to help increase your fitness level:

- Park at the farthest parking spot at the grocery store
- Walk instead of drive
- When watching the hockey game, walk in place during commercials
- Take the stairs instead of using the elevator
- Volunteer to walk the dog

Once you feel a bit stronger, feel free to start planning a specific workout routine. Start off by dedicating 5 to 10 minutes every other day to a physical activity that you enjoy. Add 5 to 10 minutes to your routine every week until you reach at least 30 minutes of moderate exercise a day. Increasing that to 60 minutes a day will be even more beneficial.

Here are some tips that will make getting started on an exercise plan easier. Once you get going, you will be surprised at how quickly you will begin to look forward to your workouts:

- Join a gym, fitness centre, YMCA or community centre. You'll have access to great facilities, and trainers and coaches who can teach you new skills to maximize your workouts.

- Plan your activity ahead of time—schedule it in your calendar. It doesn't matter what time of day you exercise. Get up with the sun and go for a walk or take a low-level aerobics class at lunchtime. If you're more of an evening person, stop by the gym an hour or two after dinner.
- Choose a variety of different activities that you enjoy or exercising will feel like a chore and you'll begin to avoid it. A good way to accomplish this is to identify activities you enjoy for each season. Walking is good all year round. In the winter, try snowshoeing or ice skating. Summer is perfect for a swim or a ride on your bike.
- Reward yourself! Whether it's indulging in a fruit smoothie on your way home from the gym or treating yourself to a live sports event after every few workouts, find a way to acknowledge your accomplishments. It will give you something to work toward beyond your physical fitness goals.

What to Ask Your Doctor If You Already Workout [SELF-HELP]

It can be hard to contemplate the possibility of losing the strength and energy you've worked so hard to build, but below are some tips that might make starting a conversation with your doctor about exercising during your illness a little bit easier.
- Start by reviewing your current fitness routine
- Discuss how much of your routine you can maintain before, during and after your treatment
- Find out if there are any new exercises you should be doing as your therapy progresses
- Ask when you can expect to be able to get back into your old routine, and come up with a plan and timeline for doing that

Exercise During Treatment

You may or may not be allowed to continue working out during your prostate cancer treatment — it all depends on the kind of therapy you're receiving.

Type of treatment	Level of exercise
Radiation therapy (external beam or brachytherapy)	You can usually continue working out during this treatment. The intensity of your activities should be based on your level of energy.
Hormone therapy	Men receiving this treatment are encouraged to exercise as they normally would.
Radical prostatectomy	Men who have received this treatment can go for leisurely walks after surgery once they are back at home— shorter, more frequent walks are recommended. Men who have had surgery should wait approximately 6 to 8 weeks before returning to more strenuous exercise, including most sports, and should avoid all heavy lifting (more than 5 kilos, or 10 pounds) for at least 6 weeks following surgery. These guidelines can also be applied to housework. Cycling should be avoided for 2 to 3 months after prostate surgery because many men say that a bicycle seat is uncomfortable. Contact sports, such as hockey, soccer and football, should be avoided for approximately 3 months.

If You Already Exercise Regularly...

If you are used to exercising regularly, it is normal to worry about the effects that your illness and treatment might have on your fitness level. You may be concerned about losing stamina and strength due to fatigue or your physical restrictions during the weeks following treatment.

Although you will have to reduce the frequency and intensity of your workouts during treatment, keep in mind that exercise has a cumulative effect. Engaging in shorter but more frequent workouts will give you similar benefits to exercising in longer but less frequent sessions.

Talk to your doctor for guidance on how best to adjust your exercise schedule during treatment or the course of your illness. You may also want to develop a plan for getting back into your regular fitness routine once your treatment is over (see Self-Help box on page 212).

Staying Motivated

If you've ever felt like you just don't want to exercise, you're not alone. Everyone at some point has trouble feeling motivated. Below are some strategies that will make it easier for you to enjoy the benefits of following a regular exercise routine.

Reason for feeling unmotivated	Strategies for staying motivated
Too busy	Exercising doesn't have to be extremely time-consuming. Find ways to incorporate exercise into your daily schedule, such as taking the stairs instead of the elevator.
Too tired	If you are tired because you are genuinely sick (e.g., with a cold), listen to your body and don't exercise. But if you are just feeling a bit low in energy after a long day, moving around will often perk you up. Do something that doesn't require a lot of concentration or effort, such as walking.
Exercise isn't fun	If you are not enjoying your exercise routine, consider changing your fitness activities or the time of day you work out. Finding a workout schedule that suits you can take a few tries, so be patient.
Lack of confidence	Get creative! Any activity that involves getting up and moving around can get your blood pumping and contribute to building your strength and endurance. It's okay to start slowly and work your way up to a more challenging workout.

Continued..

Reason for feeling unmotivated	Strategies for staying motivated
Lack of support	Although it can be fun and motivating to exercise with and have support from family and friends, keeping yourself fit is ultimately up to you and no one else. If you find that you are embarking on an exercise program with little or no support, try focusing on the positive, such as how great you feel after you work out. Remind yourself what your goals are and how working out helps you achieve them.
Lack of resources	Select activities that do not require you to take the time to develop new skills or acquire new equipment, such as walking, jogging or cycling (if you already have a bicycle).
Bad weather	There are lots of great places to exercise indoors if the weather is bad. Take a walk at a nearby mall or at your favourite museum. Go to the gym or take a fitness class at your community centre.

What Happens Next?

Exercise combined with a healthy eating plan can go a long way toward helping you prepare for and recover from your surgery. Read Chapter 11 to find out whether or not your surgery worked. You can also read more about the medications your doctor will prescribe in Chapter 16.

Chapter 15

gay men and prostate cancer

What Happens in This Chapter
- Why prostate cancer may be different for gay men
- How healthcare professionals can help
- How prostate cancer treatments impact gay sex
- Erectile difficulties and solutions
- Practical advice when seeking group support

If you have sex with other men, your experience of prostate cancer is likely to differ in several important ways from that of men who have sex only with women. There are several reasons for this, some of them simply medical and others more subtle, including social and psychological factors. Understanding how your treatment may be affected by your sexuality, and vice versa, will help you make decisions that are right for you and get the support that you deserve.

Why Is Prostate Cancer Different for Gay Men?

A diagnosis of cancer is a huge blow for anyone. Most of us want to live as long as possible and enjoy as good a quality of life as we can manage. Fear of dying, dread of pain and anguish over the pain of those we love are universal human emotions, whether we are gay or straight. So in the big, important ways, the experience of prostate cancer is similar for all men. Why, then, have we written a chapter especially for gay men?

The reality is that the prostate cancer experience does differ in several very important ways for men who have sex with other men compared with those who don't. However, in a predominantly heterosexual world the emphasis of information for prostate cancer is on the needs and concerns of the heterosexual population. Our hope is that this chapter will not only help gay men who have been diagnosed with prostate cancer, but also will increase awareness of their special needs among the professionals who care for them.

What Do We Mean by "Gay"?

Before we start, we should explain that in most places in this chapter we are using "gay" as a shorthand. If your sexual experience includes sex with other men, the advice in this chapter is for you, whether you identify yourself as gay, homosexual, bisexual, two-spirited (aboriginal), transgender or a man who has sex with men (MSM). Not all of the information will apply in your particular circumstances, so we give you the same advice as we give the heterosexual men who read the other chapters in this book: take what applies to you and leave the rest.

Working With Your Healthcare Provider

Healthcare professionals, even the most compassionate and inclusive, tend to be hetero-centred, and nowhere is this more true than in prostate cancer. One of the reasons for this is lack of scientific knowledge. Although there are over 42,000 published scientific studies on prostate cancer, remarkably there is not one single study to date specifically on prostate cancer in gay, bisexual or transgender men. This lack of scientific knowledge feeds through into medical training and the education of patient counsellors. Not surprisingly, you may find your healthcare provider is not well equipped to deal with your specific needs as a gay man.

You are thus faced with a double hit: you may be afraid to bring up your sexuality with your healthcare providers, and when you do, your physician or nurse may be unfamiliar with the issues that you face. You are not alone. Research shows that up to half of all lesbian, gay and transgender people do not disclose their sexual orientation to their healthcare team and many avoid or delay seeking care due to negative experiences related to their sexuality.

How many gay men have prostate cancer? [MORE DETAIL]

The *Canadian Community Health Survey*, conducted by Statistics Canada in 2003, found that 1.3 percent of men said they were gay. Bisexuals accounted for 0.6 percent of men. Most researchers agree these are likely underestimates, since many people are unwilling to disclose their sexuality. Canadian Cancer Statistics 2012, produced by the Canadian Cancer Society and Statistics Canada, reports that prostate cancer remains the most common cancer diagnosed in men and estimates there will be 26,500 new cases in 2012. These numbers suggest that about 500 cases will be gay/bisexual men.

When it comes to prostate cancer, this can have deadly consequences. If you avoid contact with healthcare professionals and would do anything to avoid an annual physical, a PSA test or a digital rectal exam, your prostate cancer is less likely to be detected early and may be well advanced by the time you are diagnosed. If you already have prostate cancer, keeping quiet about your sexuality means that the care you receive may not be tailored to your individual circumstances.

At least consider disclosing your sexuality to your physician or nurse. Although you may feel (quite rightly) that your sexual orientation is nobody's business, in the context of prostate cancer your sexuality is enormously relevant. There are specific health concerns that may affect gay men more than straight men (see below), and statistics on the success of the various treatments for heterosexual men may not apply to your situation and preferences. Being open about your sexuality and your feelings, thoughts, and needs will help your healthcare team do a better job of helping you and offering the most appropriate information to you in terms of maintaining your sexual health. Your sexuality is a large part of who you are. Prostate cancer will strike at the very heart of this. If you do not share your situation with your physician or nurse, he or she may be less able to help you appropriately, leaving you feeling incomplete.

Although your healthcare providers may not be able to draw on many scientific studies about gay men and prostate cancer, their role in life is to make you well and restore your quality of life, whatever that means to you personally. They have seen everything, heard everything, are sworn to secrecy and want to help you get well on your terms. If your healthcare provider is unsympathetic or uncomfortable, ask to be referred to someone who is familiar with the needs of gay men. A trusting partnership between you and your healthcare provider is a very important part of your journey when you have been diagnosed with prostate cancer.

Male Gay Sex and Prostate Cancer: Medical Issues

Erectile Dysfunction

As discussed elsewhere in this book, most treatments for prostate cancer, including radical prostatectomy (prostate surgery), radiotherapy, brachytherapy and hormone therapy, can result in either temporary or, in some cases, permanent erectile dysfunction. For a more detailed discussion of erectile dysfunction, including what you can do about it, see Chapter 13.

Although erectile dysfunction is undoubtedly one of the most dreaded consequences of prostate cancer for most men, the nature of gay sex means the effect on the penis may be less important than the effect on the rectum, depending on whether the man is a penetrator ("top") or a receiver ("bottom") or both.

For men who are solely "tops," even mild erectile dysfunction can pose sexual difficulties because it requires a stronger erection to penetrate an anus than a vagina. To have anal sex, one must pass through the strong anal sphincter muscle (which the vagina does not have). A weaker erection cannot usually pass this muscle. Even if the erection starts off strong, the act of trying to pass the anus muscle can force blood from the penis, causing it to lose rigidity. An erection that appears adequately rigid may not be firm enough for anal penetration and may require additional therapies, such as combination medication and penile rings.

No Prostate, No Pleasure?

For a man who is a "bottom," the decreased rigidity of the erection may not be as troublesome as it is for the man who is a "top." However, for "bottoms," the loss of opportunity for prostate stimulation may be an issue, since prostate cancer treatments either remove or destroy prostate tissue. The prostate is sensitive to pressure and touch, so it is an erotic zone for many men, stimulated through anal intercourse, the use of a vibrator or through perineum massage. Thus removal of the prostate may seriously alter the erotic experience, especially for men who prefer this type of stimulation.

Another consideration with prostate surgery or high doses of radiation is that there will no longer be ejaculate. For some gay men, in particular those who describe themselves as "men who have sex with men" and whose sexual experience is closely associated with the ejaculate, this may be devastating.

Bowel Side Effects

Some treatments for prostate cancer can temporarily injure the wall of the rectum, and this might seriously impair sexual function in men who are solely "bottoms."

During prostate surgery, in rare cases the wall of the rectum may be slightly damaged, although this is usually repaired right away and heals within 1 to 2 weeks. In this case, you should allow 6 to 8 weeks before having sex again.

Radiotherapy may injure the rectal wall next to the prostate, making it overly sensitive or even painful for a time. There may

221

also be some bleeding, although your physician can prescribe steroid suppositories or cortisol creams to help with this. The advice with radiotherapy is to abstain from anal intercourse for 10 to 12 weeks after treatment is finished to ensure complete healing. There is also a small possibility that the rectum may shrink after radiation treatment due to formation of scar tissue. In this case, the rectum can be gently stretched with a lubricated finger or a dilator, and your partner should proceed carefully for a while. You might also try different techniques and positions to help relax the anal sphincter.

HIV and Prostate Cancer

Life expectancy has increased over the years for men with HIV, so increasing numbers of HIV-positive men are being diagnosed with prostate cancer. We have known for many years that men with HIV are much more prone to cancer than HIV-negative men. However, a new study published in 2008 by the highly regarded US Centers for Disease Control and Prevention overturned this well-worn wisdom when it came to prostate cancer. After examining the records of over 50,000 HIV-positive men the study concluded that men with HIV are 40 percent *less* likely to be diagnosed with prostate cancer. No one is sure why this is.

More good news is that HIV status and HAART (highly active antiretroviral therapy) do not appear to make prostate cancer worse or affect how it is treated, although we still need studies that follow men over the long-term to be sure. However, whether you are HIV-positive or HIV-negative, your healthcare team will tailor your prostate cancer treatment to suit your own particular circumstances. As with any medical condition, it is important that you make the specialists who are looking after you aware of all your treatments, to ensure that all the medications work safely and effectively together.

Sex and Self-image

If you are reading this as a gay man, you will know there is great diversity in how gay men self-identify. The US Census in 2000 proved for the first time that gay, bisexual or transgender (GBT) men are a diverse group, from as many ethnic, educational, socioeconomic, cultural and geographical backgrounds as straight men. As with heterosexual men, many GBT men view themselves more in terms of their religion, cultural background, or profession, than in terms of their sexual practices.

> "A straight man may meet a woman who doesn't have a high sexual drive, but this is next to impossible in the gay world. So for many the result is growing old alone."
>
> RICHARD

However, for some gay men, especially single gay men, their sexuality, youthfulness and vitality are significant components of who they are. Their body image and their sexual lives are intertwined. "Old men's problems" like incontinence or erectile dysfunction are an especially terrifying prospect in the face of a popular culture filled with beautiful, healthy, "young" gay men. Scientific studies suggest that the search for the unrealistic ideal of male physical beauty is emerging as a serious health concern among gay men. It can lead to poor self-esteem, eating disorders, drug abuse and depression, just as it has for women. It is important for health professionals treating gay men with prostate cancer to understand this aspect of gay culture and not dismiss their patients' concerns lightly. In general, if you are becoming depressed about losing (or worrying about losing) your sexuality, your healthcare team should be able to refer you to appropriate counselling.

Dating

In general, a gay man is more likely to be single than a heterosexual man, so dating and forming intimate relationships is a very important part of his life. Many men find dating is difficult after the diagnosis of prostate cancer. Even the most confident man — gay or straight — may lose his "mojo" for a time. Some men fear the cancer itself will be an obstacle to forming new relationships, and most men dread disclosing the possibility of erection difficulties.

In particular, sexual dysfunction can seriously damage a man's ability to form new intimate relationships if those relationships are fleeting and based solely on a successful erection. This is a particular issue for MSMs, who typically have sex on the same day as the encounter. However, prostate cancer can also seriously disrupt the romantic lives of gay men seeking long-term partners.

If you are afraid to discuss your cancer because of fear of rejection, consider how you would feel if the situation were reversed. Would you shy away from someone with prostate cancer if there was an attraction there? If your date is not interested because you are a cancer survivor, or because you suffer from the side effects of prostate cancer treatments, he may not be worth getting to know in the first place.

Transgender Men

If you are a transgender male to female, the diagnosis of prostate cancer may be especially difficult for you to cope with, since you will have to live as a female diagnosed with a male cancer. If you did not have your prostate removed during your transgender operation, remember that you have the same risk for prostate cancer as other men — 1 in 7 — so you should still have an annual PSA test and digital rectal exam. We understand that these tests are not pleasant, but they could save your life. Your healthcare professional should treat you just like everyone else and be concerned only with ensuring you live a long and healthy life.

Prostate Cancer Treatment and Gay Men

The various treatments for prostate cancer have different issues for gay men than for straight men. They are described in the table on pages 226–227. These issues may be quite significant, and you and your healthcare team will need to take them into consideration when deciding on which treatment is right for you. Research is ongoing into treatments that have fewer undesirable effects such as erectile dysfunction or rectal damage. Some of the newer techniques are described on pages 188–196.

Prostate Cancer Treatments and Gay Issues

Treatment	Issues for gay men	Possible solutions

Surgery (radical prostatectomy) Open, laparoscopic or robotic (see pages 77–83)	• Nerve-sparing: temporary or permanent difficulty achieving/maintaining an erection hard enough for anal sex	• Prevention through regular stimulation of penis
		• Medication:
		  · PDE5 inhibitors
		  · Prostaglandins

	• Non-nerve-sparing: loss of erection permanent	• Vacuum devices + rings • Penile prosthesis • Prostaglandins
	• Prostate removed so decrease in sensation or loss of erotic zone	• Stimulate other erotic areas
	• No ejaculate with orgasm	• No solution

Radiation (see pages 72–75)	• Erectile dysfunction rates similar to nerve-sparing surgery
	• Complete loss of erectile function with higher doses
		• Prevention through regular stimulation of penis
		• Medication:
		  · PDE5 inhibitors
		  · Prostaglandins
		• Vacuum devices + rings
		• Penile prosthesis

	• Most of the prostate tissue is destroyed but may have some residual sensation	• Stimulate other erotic areas
	• Ejaculate gradually decreases as treatment progresses; may completely lose ejaculate, as in surgery	• No solution
	• Bowel irritation, causing increased sensitivity, pain and/or bleeding	• "Bottoms" should abstain from receiving for 10 to 12 weeks post-radiation • Steroidal suppositories • Cortisol creams
	• Bowel may lose elasticity (anal stricture), making receiving difficult	• Gentle dilation of the anus using a finger or small vibrator and "stretch" gradually

Continued

Treatment	Issues for gay men	Possible solutions

Brachytherapy (see pages 75–77)	• Erectile dysfunction rates similar to nerve-sparing surgery	• Prevention through regular stimulation of penis
		• Medication:
		  · PDE5 inhibitors
		  · Prostaglandins
		• Vacuum devices + rings
		• Penile prosthesis

	• Prostate tissue is destroyed but may have some residual sensation from areas not damaged by the implants	• Stimulate other erotic areas
	• Decreased ejaculate with orgasm	• No solution
Hormone therapy (see pages 84–86)	• Decreased libido and (usually) erectile dysfunction as for the other treatments • Achieving a hard erection may need much more stimulation	• Use more stimulation • Drugs (see above)
	• May be fatigued and lack energy • May be more depressed or moody	• Resistance training exercises help symptoms of fatigue and depression

Support for Gay Men With Prostate Cancer

This may be a time where you feel vulnerable. Past challenges and experiences may make you feel like you can cope with anything. However, this is one time where you may need to tell others how you feel and ask for support.

Regardless of sexual orientation, most men have a network of family and friends who will help them through the journey of diagnosis, treatment and recovery. Although prostate cancer can strain a relationship, romantic partners can also be a huge source of encouragement and practical help as you navigate the maze of information and recover from treatment. Anyone who cares about you will want to help, but you may need to be explicit about what you need—and pick the person for the job. Some people are comfortable discussing your worries for hour after hour; others are happiest offering practical help such as a ride from the hospital.

Support groups are lifesavers for many men and help relieve the strain on partners, who may occasionally need a break themselves (see "Resources" on page 265). Support groups for spouses are also worth considering. Even though you may feel uncomfortable at the thought of expressing your feelings to straight men and women, you will always be made to feel welcome. Some larger cities have groups especially for gay men and their partners. Prostate Cancer Canada Network has support groups for gay men as well as Side by Side groups for spouses (see www.prostatecancer.ca).

If you are not comfortable in a face-to-face setting, or you are not "out," you may find online support groups are a great alternative. Just one word of caution: be wary of online groups that offer medical advice. A good support group should offer social support only; do not follow any medical advice you receive through an online group without checking with your healthcare professional.

A Word to Healthcare Professionals

"Health promotion focuses on achieving equity in health. Health promotion action aims at reducing differences in current health status and ensuring equal opportunities and resources to enable all people to achieve their fullest health potential. This includes a secure foundation in a supportive environment..."

—The Ottawa Charter of Health Promotion, 1986

When we started to write this chapter and began researching prostate cancer in gay men, we were embarrassed to realize how little attention the medical world has paid to the subject.

Prostate cancer affects all men, without making distinctions between gay and straight. Healthcare professionals should be similarly inclusive. Everyone deserves to be treated with respect and understanding, regardless of sexual orientation. Respecting diversity is more than just an official mandate. It is very important that, as healthcare professionals, we channel both our verbal and body language to create an atmosphere of care, openness and non-judgment. We all know that the best treatment is patient-centred care—care that results from a trusting partnership between professionals and patients. In prostate cancer, understanding the role that sexuality plays in a man's quality of life is key to good management. A sensitive and informed approach is required. No longer can we accept the motto, "if we don't ask, we won't need to know."

Talking about sex isn't easy for most people, even professionals. Here's how you could open the discussion to allow patients to decide when and if to talk about their sexuality:
• What concerns do you have about your prostate surgery?
• Are you single/do you have a partner?
• How is your partner dealing with your diagnosis?
• What concerns does your partner have?

Chapter 16

medications

What Happens in This Chapter

- Hormone treatments for prostate cancer
- Medications before surgery
- General anesthetics
- Drugs after surgery
- Drugs for treating incontinence and erectile dysfunction
- Side effects

If you decide that surgery is not an option for your prostate disease, your physician can draw on a wide range of drugs to help you. If surgery is the next step, medications will play an important part in your hospital visit and afterward, from the drugs that prepare you for your procedure to those that help you recover from the aftereffects. You are the most important member of your own care team, and never more so than when it comes to medications. You should always be clear on why you are taking each medicine, how to take it correctly and any possible side effects, so that you can help your physician find the best combination for you.

Medications for Cancer

Prostate cancer is not primarily treated with "conventional" chemotherapy cancer drugs. The idea behind most drug treatments for prostate cancer is to "starve" prostate cancer cells of the hormone testosterone, because these cells need testosterone to grow and develop. Although these medications do not eradicate the cancer entirely, they can shrink the tumour and suppress the cancer very effectively. The three groups of hormonal drugs that shrink prostate cancer are LHRH agonists, LHRH antagonists and antiandrogens. Because these drugs are an important alternative to surgery, they are discussed in detail in Chapter 5 (pages 92–95).

When hormone therapy doesn't work, chemotherapy with a drug called docetaxel (Taxotere) can be effective (see page 95).

Medications Before Surgery

Anemia Therapy

If you are anemic before surgery, for several weeks beforehand you may be given iron tablets, vitamins (e.g., B12 or folate) or injections of synthetic erythropoietin (e.g., epoetin alfa), a hormone that stimulates your body to make more red blood cells. After radical prostatectomy, you may be given iron tablets for a few months to help your hemoglobin levels recover faster.

Stool Softeners/Laxatives

Before your operation you may be prescribed a stronger laxative or enema to cleanse your bowels in preparation for surgery.

These may include colonic washout preparations such as Golytely, Klean-Prep or Colyte. Other solutions used include magnesium citrate (Citro-Mag or Royvac). Some hospitals may recommend a Fleet enema as well.

Once you're in the hospital for your surgery, you'll be given some new types of medication that each serve a different purpose: sedatives, deep vein thrombosis (DVT) prophylaxis and antibiotics.

Sedatives
Your anesthesiologist may give you a sedative right before you're taken to the operating room. The purpose of a sedative is to help you feel more relaxed.

DVT Prophylaxis
To decrease the chances of developing a blood clot during or after your surgery, you will be given a blood-thinning medication (e.g., heparin) through an injection with a very small needle. You will usually have this medication twice a day after your surgery until you are discharged from the hospital.

Antibiotics
You will also receive antibiotics intravenously (through a vein) before your operation, to prevent infection during and after surgery. These antibiotics will be continued for about 24 hours (depending on your hospital's protocol) after your operation. You may also be given a prescription for antibiotic pills to take home as a special precaution for when the catheter is removed. Antibiotic ointments such as Polysporin may also be used around the catheter insertion site. It's important to tell your doctor or nurse if you're allergic to any antibiotics.

Medications During Surgery

For a radical prostatectomy you will almost certainly receive a **general anesthetic**. General anesthetics, which are given intravenously and as a gas, do more than just put you to sleep. They also help with pain control, relax your muscles and cause amnesia (loss of memory), allowing you to forget events immediately before and after your surgery.

The dosing for your anesthetic will be carefully calculated and adjusted based on your age, weight, past medical history and anticipated length of surgery. During surgery your anesthesiologist will make careful adjustments to your general anesthetic, based on how you are responding. When you wake up you may experience side effects such as nausea, vomiting, disorientation and headache, although this is relatively uncommon. If they happen to you, they can be effectively treated and should go away within the first 24 hours after surgery.

General anesthetics have evolved greatly since they were first used. There is now a wide variety of different anesthetic drugs that provide a more controllable and safer kind of general anesthetic experience. The stages of anesthesia can be broken down into **induction**, **maintenance**, **reversal** and **recovery**.

Induction is the period when you are "put to sleep," most commonly with an intravenous drug. The maintenance period covers the time when the actual surgery takes place. Your anesthesiologist uses a combination of drugs to keep you asleep, relaxed and pain free, either through your mask or intravenously. During reversal, special drugs are used to reverse the effects of anesthesia and wake you up. During the recovery phase, you are monitored closely to make sure that all is well as you wake up.

Medications After Your Surgery

Pain Relievers

After your surgery you will be given pain relief medication such as the anti-inflammatory drug ketorolac (Toradol) or acetaminophen (Tylenol). A narcotic such as morphine is sometimes given in addition to these painkillers (although narcotics are becoming increasingly uncommon). Pain control is an important part of your hospital stay, so it is covered in detail in Chapter 9.

Drugs for Bladder Spasm

Some men may experience bladder spasms while the catheter is in place after surgery due to the catheter irritating the muscles of the bladder. The spasm may feel like a strong urge to pee, or you may experience actual pain. There are a number of drugs that can help with this, including anticholinergic drugs such as oxybutynin (Ditropan) or tolterodine (Detrol) taken by mouth, and opium and belladonna suppositories administered into the rectum. Medication for bladder spasms should be stopped 24 hours before the catheter is removed. Side effects of these drugs may include blurred vision, drowsiness and dry mouth.

Antiemetics

Some of the medications you receive for controlling your pain after surgery may cause nausea and vomiting. There are a number of drugs available to help with this, such as dimenhydrinate (Gravol), prochlorperazine (Stemetil) and granisetron (Kytril), which can be taken orally or given through your intravenous line. Side effects of these drugs may include dizziness, drowsiness and dry mouth.

Stool Softeners/Laxatives

Stool softeners such as docusate sodium (Colace) are prescribed after surgery to prevent constipation. A number of factors, such as a low-fibre diet, immobilization, pain control drugs and the surgery itself, can cause constipation. Laxatives, which work by increasing the motion of the bowels, may be prescribed for you to take for 1 to 2 weeks once you are home. These may include sennosides (Senokot).

Medications for Incontinence

Medications designed to help reduce bladder spasm — oxybutynin and tolterodine — can also reduce leakage and the frequent, urgent need to urinate, if this is caused by an overactive bladder. The side effects of these drugs — symptoms such as dry mouth, blurred vision and palpitations — appear to be less common with tolterodine. They also cannot be used in people with any type of bladder obstruction, so they are not suitable for men with enlarged prostates and are also ineffective for incontinence after radical prostatectomy in most men.

Medications for Erectile Dysfunction

Erectile dysfunction drugs fall into two main categories: those that rapidly create an erection (e.g., MUSE and Caverject) and those that allow an erection to happen if you are sexually stimulated (e.g., Cialis, Levitra, Staxyn, Viagra). There drugs are covered in detail in Chapter 13.

Antihistamines

Some of the medications you receive for controlling your pain may cause itching and possible hives or rash. There are a number of drugs available to help with this, such as diphenhydramine (Benadryl) or loratadine (Claritin). These may be taken orally, or Benadryl may be given through your intravenous line.

Medications and Potential Side Effects

Drugs	Common side effects
Medications for benign prostate disease	
Alpha-blockers	
e.g., alfuzosin (Xatral), doxazosin (Cardura), tamsulosin (Flomax), terazosin (Hytrin)	Dizziness or faintness after rising from a lying or sitting position, headaches, nausea, heart palpitations, stuffy nose, tiredness or weakness, diarrhea, rash
	Xatral: possible angina and dry mouth
	Hytrin: abnormal ejaculation
	RARELY—heart failure and stroke
5-alpha-reductase inhibitors	
e.g., finasteride (Proscar), dutasteride (Avodart)	Erectile dysfunction, loss of libido, ejaculation disorder, breast enlargement (gynecomastia)
Hormones for prostate cancer	
LHRH agonists/antagonists	
e.g., goserelin (Zoladex), leuprolide (Eligard, Lupron, Trelstar), degeralix (Firmagon)	Hot flashes, sweating, erectile dysfunction, shrinkage of testicles, rash, injection site pain/redness, breast enlargement (gynecomastia), headache
Antiandrogens	
e.g., bicalutamide (Casodex), flutamide (Euflex)	Casodex: hot flashes, itching, dry skin (pruritus), breast tenderness, breast enlargement (gynecomastia), diarrhea, nausea, vomiting, weakness
	Euflex: breast enlargement (gynecomastia), breast tenderness, flow of milk from breast (galactorrhea)
Chemotherapy for prostate cancer	
Docetaxel (Taxotere)	Nausea, vomiting, lethargy, increased risk of infection, lower white blood counts

Continued..

Medications and Potential Side Effects

Drugs	Common side effects
Medications for surgery	
Anemia therapy	
e.g., synthetic erythropoietins: epoetin alfa (Eprex), darbepoetin alfa (Aranesp); iron tablets: ferrous fumarate, ferrous gluconate, ferrous sulfate	Erythropoietin: chest pain, edema, rash, itching, diarrhea, injection site redness, heart problems, infections, nausea, high or low blood pressure
	Iron tablets: constipation, diarrhea
Antibiotics	
e.g., ampicillin, ciprofloxacin, clindamycin, gentamycin, cotrimoxazole, Polysporin ointment, Neosporin ointment	Diarrhea, oral thrush, nausea, vomiting, stomach cramps, skin rash, kidney problems (gentamycin)
Anticoagulants	
e.g., heparin (Hepalean), warfarin (Coumadin), LMWH, dalteparin (Fragmin)	Pain, bruising at injection site, fever, skin eruptions, decreased platelet count
Antiemetics	
e.g., dimenhydrinate (Gravol), granisetron (Kytril), prochlorperazine (Stemetil)	Dimenhydrinate: drowsiness, dizziness, dry mouth
	Prochlorperazine: nervous symptoms, twitching, tremor, shaking
	Granisetron: headache, weakness, fatigue, constipation or diarrhea
Antihistamines	
e.g., diphenhydramine (Benadryl), loratadine (Claritin)	drowsiness, possible decrease in urine flow
Drugs for bladder spasms	
e.g., opium and belladonna suppositories, oxybutynin (Ditropan), tolterodine (Detrol)	Dry mouth, blurred vision, dry skin, constipation, drowsiness, heart beat irregularities, nausea
General anesthetics	
e.g., midazolam (Versed), fentanyl (Sublimaze), nitrous oxide	Nausea, vomiting, disorientation, headache for up to 24 hours

Continued...

Medications and Potential Side Effects

Drugs	Common side effects
Pain relievers	
e.g., Non-narcotics: ketorolac (Toradol), acetaminophen (regular Tylenol)	Ketorolac: stomach and intestinal bleeding
Narcotics: acetaminophen + codeine (Tylenol), acetaminophen + oxycodone (Percocet), morphine	Narcotics: dizziness, lightheadedness, nausea, vomiting, dry mouth, constipation, drowsiness, disorientation, skin rash, sweating, low blood pressure, shallow breathing
Steroids and suppositories: creams such as Anusol HC cream and suppositories	
Bowel routine	
e.g., bisacodyl (Dulcolax), docusate sodium (Colace), sennosides (Senokot), Fleet enema, Colyte, Golytely, Klean-Prep, Citro-Mag, Royvac	Abdominal discomfort, nausea, diarrhea
Incontinence therapy	
Urinary antispasmotics	
e.g., oxybutynin (Ditropan), tolterodine (Detrol)	Dry mouth, blurred vision, dry skin, itching, constipation or diarrhea, drowsiness, heart palpitations, nausea
Erectile dysfunction therapy	
PDE5 inhibitors	
e.g., tadalafil (Cialis), vardenafil (Levitra), vardenafil orally disintegrating tablet (Staxyn), sildenafil (V6iagra)	Headache, flushing, gastrointestinal upset, nasal congestion
	RARELY—loss of hearing, blindness
Prostaglandins	
e.g., alprostadil (MUSE, Caverject)	Bruising (Caverject), penile pain, prolonged erection (4 hours or more)

Coping With Side Effects

All drugs have the potential to cause side effects. The goal is to avoid side effects or keep them to a minimum. Your physician can also prescribe or recommend extra medication to help you cope with some of them. For example, he or she may suggest stool softeners or laxatives (see above) to deal with the constipation that comes with pain-relieving medication. Increasing the dose of a drug gradually often reduces the risk of side effects. To find out more about the downsides of your drugs, read the information that comes with your medication or ask your pharmacist or physician.

What Happens Next?

It's surprising how many people don't fill their prescriptions for medications that can make a huge difference to their health. If you have concerns about something your doctor has prescribed, or if you find that a drug is giving you side effects, talk to your physician. Maintaining open communication with your medical team will ensure that you receive the best treatment available.

Chapter 17

future directions in prostate cancer treatment

What Happens in This Chapter
- Taking part in a clinical trial
- High-intensity focused ultrasound that "cooks" the prostate
- MRI targeted focal therapy

Prostate cancer treatment is always evolving, and patients today can benefit from advances that have already taken place, as well as help spur on further improvements by taking part in clinical trials. Future technologies aim to maintain the excellent cure rates seen for surgery and radiation while reducing side effects such as erectile dysfunction and urinary incontinence.

Clinical Trials and You

The key to all new medical advances is clinical research—research on real people. The purpose of clinical research trials is to find out whether a particular medication, device or technique is both effective and safe. Canadian hospitals are renowned worldwide for excellence in conducting clinical trials. If you are eligible to take part in any of these studies, you will be helping to test new treatments and playing a direct role in providing new options for treating prostate disease in Canada.

Clinical trials may be sponsored by a pharmaceutical company, biotechnology company or government agency, but all trials must be officially approved by the hospital and independent ethics review boards before a study can begin. In most trials, neither patients nor researchers know until the end of the trial which patients are receiving the treatment itself or a placebo (non-active treatment). The advantage of this "double-blind" approach is that the results are non-biased. The disadvantage for patients is that they may not receive the new therapy—they may find themselves in the placebo group—or the new therapy may prove to be ineffective.

If you have prostate cancer, you may be offered the chance to test a new drug that fights prostate cancer before surgery or improves treatment afterward. Even better, you may be asked to participate in a study evaluating a new curative treatment for prostate cancer. Your physician will determine whether you are eligible for a clinical trial and approach you to take part; however, the decision is always yours. If you are not interested, it will not affect the quality of your care in any way.

If you are interested in getting involved in a clinical research trial, your best bet is to ask your physician. The National

Cancer Institute or Canadian Cancer Society Research Institute
are other good resources for information about clinical trials
involving patients like you.

New Advances in Prostate Cancer Treatment

High-Intensity Focused Ultrasound (HIFU)

HIFU has been around for many years but has only recently
been used for treating prostate cancer. The concept behind this
new treatment is, in effect, to "cook" the prostate gland while
minimizing collateral damage to the surrounding healthy tissues.
A high-intensity ultrasound beam inserted into the rectum
simultaneously melts the prostate (by heating it to 85 C [185 F]
or more) and creates an image of the prostate gland and
surrounding tissues in real time. Ultrasound technology—best
known for taking pictures of unborn babies—is actually quite
old and has been around since the early part of the 20th century.
However, only recently has it been safely reinvented for prostate
cancer treatment.

One of the major pluses of HIFU is that, although it requires a
general or a spinal anesthetic, it requires no incision, so men go
home the same day and recover quickly. A catheter is still needed
afterward, like the ones used after radical prostatectomy. Some
men also require a catheter that comes out of the lower end of
the abdomen (called a suprapubic catheter).

The other appeal of HIFU is that it seems to have minimal effect
on the erection nerves and the muscles for urinary control.
Studies so far show that men who had HIFU were much less

likely to have erectile dysfunction or urinary incontinence than men who had undergone surgery or radiation treatment.

However, before you stampede toward HIFU, take note that physicians still need convincing that HIFU is as good at curing cancer as surgery or radiation treatment. Cancer centres in Europe, which have the longest experience with HIFU (10 years to date) have reported that HIFU appears to be less effective at controlling cancer than surgery.

Another downside with HIFU is that, although incontinence is less of a problem, other types of urinary problems might show up afterward. A rare medical complication of HIFU is a recto-urethral fistula. In this disorder a "tunnel" develops between the rectum and the urethra, so men end up passing urine through the rectum and vice versa. This complication is almost unheard of with surgery or radiation. Some men have also developed a severe blockage in the urethra at the site of the "melted" prostate, causing urinary retention. This is why some doctors who perform HIFU install the suprapubic catheter as a backup drainage device.

Finally, bear in mind that HIFU is still very much an experimental procedure. The US Food and Drug Administration (FDA), for example, has not yet approved HIFU for use in the US, although it is approved in Canada.

If you're still interested in HIFU, how can you get it? It is not covered by public health insurance in Canada, so you would have to pay for it yourself. As with all therapies, especially new ones, you should have a detailed discussion with your urologist to determine whether HIFU is right for you, given its risks and benefits.

MRI Targeted Focal Laser Therapy

Similar to HIFU, other forms of focal therapy are in their experimental stages. The most promising is the use of **magnetic resonance imaging (MRI)** to help direct treatment to specific areas of the prostate where the cancer is located. By locating and treating the cancer cells only, normal cells of the prostate are spared, minimizing side effects, particularly incontinence and erectile dysfunction. This is a day procedure utilizing a mild general anesthetic. Men walk out of the hospital with a Foley catheter in place and return a few days later to have it removed.

As appealing as it sounds, this is still an experimental procedure, and it is unclear whether applying focal therapy is sufficient for curing prostate cancer. Prostate cancer is notoriously known as a multi-focal disease. This means that the cancer is located in many different areas of the prostate gland—some you can see with medical imaging and some you can't. Thus, research studies will be needed before we can conclude whether applying focal therapy is as effective as the conventional treatments of surgery or radiation.

Chapter 18

who's who of hospital staff

What Happens in This Chapter
- Hospital staff you will meet
- A brief description of their roles

When you go into the hospital, you will encounter a large number of staff. In general, they will be friendly and helpful. If you are dealing with them directly, they should introduce themselves and explain their roles to you.

However, it can be confusing that many of the hospital staff, from porters to doctors, wear white coats or "scrubs" (loose pants and tops of different colours), making it hard to figure out who's who. Also, within the title of "doctor" or "nurse" are a number of different roles, making it difficult to understand what each of these people does. For example, you may see a **fellow**, a **resident** or a **staff physician**. All are doctors, but they have varying levels of knowledge, ability and responsibility. Or, you may see a **ward nurse**, a **recovery room nurse** or a **research nurse**. Again, all are qualified nurses, but each has a different role.

This chapter will give you a brief overview explaining who is who in the hospital and each person's role in your care.

[MORE DETAIL]

Medical Staff	Nursing Staff	Support Staff
Anesthesiologist	Community care	Anesthesia technician
Fellow	access coordinator/	Blood technician
Medical student	homecare nurse	Chaplain/pastor/priest
Oncologist	Nurse practitioner	Clerk
Pathologist	Registered nurse	Dietitian
Psychologist	Research nurse	ECG technician
Radiologist		Patient care assistant/
Resident		orderly/nurse's aide
Surgeon		Physiotherapist
		Volunteer

Anesthesia Technician

A person who is trained to assist the anesthesiologist in caring for a patient while the patient is under anesthesia.

Anesthesiologist

A doctor who administers anesthesia to reduce or eliminate pain and put surgery patients to sleep. The anesthesiologist's job includes medically evaluating patients before surgery, consulting with the surgical team, providing pain control, supporting life during surgery, making decisions about blood conservation and transfusions, supervising care after surgery, and discharging patients from the recovery unit or the intensive care unit.

Blood Technician

A person qualified to take blood from patients.

Chaplain/Pastor/Priest

A person who is ordained to be a religious leader. He or she can provide counselling, prayer and last rites for patients. The chaplain may be non-denominational.

Clerk

This is usually the first person you will meet when you arrive at the ward. He or she is responsible for answering the phone in the ward, but his or her role often extends beyond this, depending on experience level.

Community Care Access Coordinator/Homecare Nurse

In some hospitals, this nurse will work with your community and coordinate your care after you're discharged from the hospital.

Dietitian

This professional assists the healthcare team with recommendations regarding a patient's diet. A dietitian's advice is especially important for the team caring for people with diabetes and those with special food restrictions.

ECG Technician
A person who is specifically trained to perform ECGs on patients.

Fellow
A fully qualified doctor who has specialized in a particular area of medicine or surgery, usually with a few years of experience. Fellows can come from other countries to spend up to 3 years gaining additional experience.

Medical Student
A person who is enrolled in medical school and is being trained to become a medical doctor.

Nurse Practitioner
A registered nurse who has completed a master's degree in nursing. He or she performs advanced physical examinations and takes patients' medical histories. The nurse practitioner is also responsible for the coordination of patient care and patient education and works both independently and in collaboration with the healthcare team in making rounds, ordering diagnostic tests, interpreting the results and deciding on treatment.

Oncologist
A doctor who specializes in the treatment and management of cancer. He or she may be a radiologist, internist or surgeon who has had further specialized training.

Pathologist
A doctor who specializes in examining and analyzing tissue samples under a microscope. This is the person who assigns the Gleason score to tumours.

Patient Care Assistant/Orderly/Nurse's Aide

A trained member of the healthcare team who provides patient care under the supervision of a nurse. He or she may be the one to accompany you to tests or procedures.

Physiotherapist

Someone who is trained to work with patients to improve their physical function, endurance, coordination and range of motion. Physiotherapy for prostate surgery patients can include physical exercise, coughing and deep breathing.

Psychologist

A trained professional (usually with a PhD) who specializes in clinical counselling. The psychologist helps guide those who are having difficulty in adjusting to an event that alters their lives — in this case the diagnosis of prostate cancer.

Radiologist

A doctor who specializes in reading radiological tests, such as X-rays, ultrasounds and CAT scans.

Registered Nurse

The nurse who is usually primarily responsible for your basic care. Helps to coordinate, plan and assess your needs throughout your surgical experience. He or she works closely with your surgeon. In bigger teaching centres, in particular, nurses may function in different capacities, such as a recovery room (PACU) nurse, operating room nurse, educator, coordinator or nurse manager.

Research Nurse

A nurse, usually with a university degree, who specializes in assisting and coordinating research. It is his or her job to approach patients for possible participation in research studies and coordinate their involvement. In some instances, the research nurse is also responsible for collecting blood samples for the studies and will see participants at follow-up appointments.

Resident
A physician who has completed medical school and is undergoing specialized training. He or she can specialize in a particular area, such as surgery or oncology (cancer care). If you are having your surgery at a university-affiliated hospital, you will encounter many residents. Although they are still in training, residents are certified physicians and are considered front-line workers. They take 24-hour-call shifts and are just minutes away if an emergency arises. At teaching hospitals, in particular, they are vital to excellent patient care.

Surgeon
A doctor who specializes in performing surgery. Your urologist performs your surgery with the assistance of a resident and supervises your care before and after surgery.

Volunteer
A person who donates his or her time to the hospital. He or she may have one of a wide variety of roles.

Disclaimer
The above descriptions are intended as a general guide only. The roles of each type of staff member mentioned may differ slightly from hospital to hospital.

glossary

Acute normovolemic hemodilution Some of your own blood is taken at the time of surgery and returned to your body at the end of surgery.

Adenocarcinoma The most common type of prostate cancer.

Adjuvant treatment Treatment given to patients after surgery to kill remaining cancer cells (if the pathology is positive) and to reduce the chances of cancer returning. Chemotherapy and radiation are adjuvant, or additional, treatments following surgery.

Analgesic A medication that relieves pain.

Androgen A hormone, such as testosterone, that promotes male characteristics such as sexual function and muscle mass.

Anemia A lower than normal level of hemoglobin in the blood.

Anesthetic A drug used to numb an area of skin ("local") or put someone to sleep ("general"). Radical prostatectomy is usually done under general anesthetic, which means you are completely asleep and will not feel any pain. If you are having surgery for benign prostatic hyperplasia (not cancer), you may be given the option of a spinal anesthetic, which means you will be numbed from the waist down but will remain awake.

Antiandrogen Any compound that blocks the effects of androgens, or male hormones.

251

Antibiotics Medications used to treat or prevent infections.

Anticholinergics Medications used to help relax the bladder muscle in order to reduce bladder spasms.

Antiemetics Medications taken to help prevent or reduce nausea.

Antihistamines Medications used to help decrease itching and swelling from an allergic reaction.

Antioxidants Chemicals that reduce the damaging effects of oxygen on tissues.

Anus The lowest part of the bowel that exits the body and allows defecation.

Artificial sphincter A device used to replace a damaged or removed urinary sphincter.

ASAP *See* Atypical small acinar cell proliferation

Atherosclerosis A condition where fatty plaques block the arteries.

Atypical small acinar cell proliferation (ASAP) A diagnosis where cells could be cancerous. Further tests are required for confirmation.

Autologous blood donation Your own blood is collected and stored before surgery. In the event that you need a blood transfusion, your own blood can be used rather than a donor's.

Benign Non-cancerous, or non-malignant.

Benign prostatic hyperplasia (BPH) Non-cancerous growth of the prostate that happens in many men as they age. Occasionally called benign prostatic hypertrophy.

BPH *See* Benign prostatic hyperplasia.

Biopsy A tissue sample taken from your prostate and checked under a microscope in order to help make a diagnosis.

Bladder The muscular, sack-like organ that stores urine

until it can be released from your body.

Bladder neck The opening of the bladder into the urethra.

Bone scan A nuclear medicine test that is performed to see bones. It can detect abnormalities such as arthritis, fractures and cancer.

Brachytherapy A type of radiation treatment. Radioactive seeds are implanted in your prostate to kill surrounding tissue, including cancer cells.

Cancer Abnormal cells that grow uncontrollably.

Carcinoma A cancerous tumour that originates in an organ such as the prostate.

Castration Removing the testicles with surgery, or using medication to stop the testes from functioning. Castration lowers testosterone levels to near zero.

CAT scan *See* Computerized axial tomography (CAT) scan.

Catheter A narrow, flexible tube that is inserted into a part of the body, usually to drain fluids.

Central line (CL) An intravenous catheter that is placed in your neck.

Chemotherapy Using pharmaceutical drugs to treat cancer.

Clinical staging A process where the doctor estimates the size of the cancer and whether it has spread.

Clinical trials Carefully planned studies that evaluate new or experimental treatments, or existing treatments for different types of patients.

Computerized axial tomography (CAT) scan A painless medical test that helps physicians make a diagnosis. CAT scans use X-ray equipment to produce images of the inside of your body and computers to combine those images and generate cross-sectional and 3D views.

Constriction ring A ring or band that is placed at the base of the penis to maintain an erection.

Corpus cavernosum One of two chambers that run the length of the penis and fill with blood to produce an erection.

Corpus spongiosum A spongy chamber in the penis, near the urethra, that leads to the head of the penis. It fills with blood to help produce an erection.

Creatinine A waste product that is tested to see how well your kidneys are functioning.

Cryotherapy A form of treatment for prostate cancer. Liquid nitrogen is used to freeze the prostate gland and kill tissue, including cancer cells.

Cystoscopy A procedure performed by a urologist so that he or she can see inside the urethra, bladder and prostate, using a scope inserted through the urethra.

Deep vein thrombosis (DVT) A blood clot in one or more veins deep in the body.

Detrusor The muscle layer that surrounds the bladder and allows it to contract when you urinate.

Digital rectal exam (DRE) An examination of the prostate. Your physician inserts a lubricated gloved finger into the rectum to feel for abnormalities in the prostate.

Dihydrotestosterone (DHT) A powerful hormone derived from testosterone that could be needed by prostate cancer cells to grow.

Diverticula Pockets of tissue that have grown on the bladder and can trap urine.

DHT See Dihydrotestosterone.

Dorsal venous complex Important blood vessels that sit directly on top of the prostate.

DRE *See* Digital rectal exam.

254

DVT *See* Deep vein thrombosis.

Ejaculation The release of semen from the penis during orgasm.

Electrolytes Substances in our bodies that are essential for healthy function of cells and organs. They are measured to assess body systems, such as normal or abnormal kidney function.

Epididymis Coiled tubes that are located behind the testicles and that store sperm until they are matured.

Epidural A small, thin tube, placed in the spine, through which medication can be given. Used for anesthesia and pain management.

Estrogen A female sex hormone.

Erectile dysfunction A problem in achieving and maintaining an erection.

External beam radiotherapy Radiation treatment for prostate cancer using high-energy X-rays.

Foley catheter A tube inserted through the urethra to drain urine from the bladder.

Frenum or frenulum The small v-shaped tissue that connects the glans of the penis to the foreskin; also known as the man's G-spot.

Free PSA PSA that is not bound to proteins in the blood.

Free radicals Unstable molecules that can damage cells in the body.

Glans The cap-shaped tip of the penis.

Gleason Grading System A scoring system commonly used to describe how aggressive prostate cancer is.

Hematuria Blood in the urine.

Hemoglobin The part of the red blood cell that carries oxygen.

Hemolytic reaction A negative reaction to a blood transfusion.

Hesitancy Difficulty in starting urine flow.

HIFU *See* High-intensity focused ultrasound.

High-intensity focused ultrasound (HIFU) A medical treatment that uses extreme heat generated by ultrasound waves to destroy tissue.

Hormone A chemical that is produced in one organ of the body and travels through the bloodstream to trigger the function of another organ.

Hormone-refractory prostate cancer Prostate cancer that has stopped responding to hormone therapy.

Hot spots Abnormalities that show up on a bone scan and may be arthritis, previous bone fractures or tumours.

IM *See* Intramuscular.

Impotence When you are unable to achieve or maintain an erection.

Incision A cut made by the surgeon during surgery.

Incontinence Partial or total loss of urinary control. There are different types of incontinence, such as stress incontinence and urge incontinence.

Intensity-modulated radiation therapy (IMRT) A form of external radiation treatment in which the dose is highly concentrated on the tumour. This increases the effectiveness of the treatment and decreases damage to surrounding areas.

Internal sphincter The muscular ring-like band of the bladder neck that retains urine in the bladder until you release it.

Intramuscular (IM) Injected into the muscle.

Intravenous (IV) Injected into a vein.

IMRT *See* Intensity-modulated radiation therapy.

IV *See* Intravenous.

Jackson–Pratt drain A device with a bulb and a tube used to drain excess fluid from the surgery site. It is usually removed a day or two after surgery.

Kegel exercises Pelvic muscle exercises you can do to help strengthen muscles that control urination.

Laparoscopic radical prostatectomy (LRP) Surgery to remove the prostate that is performed through small incisions, using small, telescope-like instruments.

LHRH *See* Luteinizing hormone-releasing hormone

Libido Sexual desire or sex drive.

LRP *See* Laparoscopic radical prostatectomy

Luteinizing hormone-releasing hormone (LHRH) agonist or antagonist A medication used to suppress the body's production of male hormones.

Lymph nodes Clusters of grape-shaped tissues that help defend the body against infections. They are found throughout the body (e.g., in the groin, neck and underarms).

Magnetic resonance imaging (MRI) A test that uses magnetic and radio waves to produce detailed pictures of organs inside the body.

Malignant Cancerous.

Margins The cut edge of tissue that is removed during surgery. A "positive" surgical margin means that cancer cells are visible at the outer edge of the removed tissue, indicating that cancer cells may remain in the body. A "negative" margin means that no cancer cells are visible, which may indicate there are no cancer cells left behind in the body.

Meatus The opening of the urethra at the head of the penis.

Metastasis Spread of cancer beyond where it originated. Prostate cancer tends to spread to the lymph nodes and bones.

MRI *See* Magnetic resonance imaging.

Narcotics Medications used to control pain, such as morphine, Demerol, Percocet, Percodan or Tylenol with codeine.

Nerve grafting Replacing a nerve that was removed during prostatectomy with a healthy nerve from another part of the body.

Nerve-sparing A type of prostatectomy in which the surgeon spares, or saves, the nerves that control erections.

Nocturia A need to urinate frequently during the night.

Non-steroidal anti-inflammatory drug (NSAID) A medication used to relieve pain and inflammation.

NSAID *See* Non-steroidal anti-inflammatory drug.

Oncologist A doctor who specializes in treating cancer.

Open radical prostatectomy (ORP) The traditional approach to prostate removal. The surgeon removes the prostate by hand with standard surgical instruments.

Orchiectomy The surgical removal of one or both of the testicles.

ORP *See* Open radical prostatectomy.

Orgasm Sexual climax.

Pathological staging Tissu samples removed during surgery or biopsy are examined under a microscope to determine the stage, or extent, of the cancer.

Pathologist A doctor who specializes in examining tissue samples, for example, looking for the presence of cancer cells and information about those cells.

Penile implant A treatment option for men who are not able to achieve an erection. A prosthesis that enables erections is surgically implanted in the penis.

Penis The male organ for urination and sexual intercourse.

Perineum The area between the scrotum and anus.

Peroxides Molecules that can sometimes break down into free radicals and damage cells in the body.

Phosphodiesterase-5 (PDE5) inhibitors Medications used to treat erectile dysfunction. Cialis, Levitra, Staxyn and Viagra are all PDE5 inhibitors.

PIN *See* Prostatic intraepithelial neoplasia.

PIV *See* Peripheral intravenous line.

Placebo A non-active and safe substance that is often used as the basis for comparisons with drug treatments in clinical trials.

Priapism An erection that lasts for longer than 4 hours and is considered an urgent medical condition needing treatment.

Prognosis A doctor's prediction of how a patient's cancer will progress, and the chances for recovery.

Prostaglandin therapy A treatment for erectile dysfunction.

Prostate A walnut-sized gland that is located below the bladder and surrounds the urethra. The prostate produces the fluid that combines with semen when you ejaculate.

Prostatic intraepithelial neoplasia (PIN) Once thought to be a precursor to prostate cancer, but this is no longer the case.

Prostatic specific antigen (PSA) A protein produced by the prostate gland. PSA is measured in blood tests to detect potential problems in the prostate. High PSA levels could mean the presence of prostate cancer.

Prostatitis Inflammation or infection of the prostate.

PSA velocity (PSAV) The rate at which PSA changes over time.

PSAD *See* PSA density.

PSAV *See* PSA velocity.

Radical prostatectomy Surgery to completely remove the prostate and the tissue surrounding it.

Radiologist A doctor who specializes in reading and interpreting X-rays, CAT scans and other radiological tests.

RALRP *See* Robot-assisted laparoscopic radical prostatectomy

Randomized clinical trial The design preferred by the medical community for doing a scientific study. Researchers randomly assign participants to a treatment group or no treatment group.

Rectum The lowest part of bowel that connects to the anus.

Resectoscope A long, thin telescopic device that the surgeon inserts through the urethra to remove tissue from the prostate.

Retrograde ejaculation Semen flows up into the bladder, instead of exiting via the urethra, during ejaculation. This is due to damage to the bladder neck and happens frequently after transurethral resection of the prostate (TURP).

Robot-assisted laparoscopic radical prostatectomy

(RALRP) Robot-assisted surgery to remove the prostate through small incisions in the abdomen. Small, telescope-like instruments provide a 3D view of the surgical area.

Salvage treatment A procedure designed to "rescue" a patient when a previous treatment fails and the cancer returns.

Saturation biopsy A larger number of samples of prostate tissue are taken in this procedure than in the usual biopsy. The patient is usually given a general anesthetic.

Scrotum The sack that hangs behind the penis and contains the testicles.

Semen A whitish fluid released at ejaculation that contains sperm and other fluids.

Seminal vesicles Small glands that are connected to the prostate and excrete fluid into the semen during ejaculation.

Stage A measure of whether the cancer has spread outside the prostate.

Staples A method of closing an incision; they may be used inside the body, as well.

Stent A thin, flexible tube used to support body "tubes" such as an artery or the urethra.

Stress incontinence The involuntary leaking of urine during activities that increase pressure on the abdomen, such as coughing, laughing, lifting heavy objects or exercising.

Sutures Surgical stitching used to close an incision. Sutures may be dissolvable or non-dissolvable.

Testes, or testicles Part of the male genitals that produce sperm and testosterone. They are located in the scrotum, behind the penis.

Testosterone The primary male sex hormone, or androgen, that is responsible for developing and maintaining men's sex drive and sexual function as well as muscle mass and strength. It may encourage the growth of prostate cancer.

Transition zone Innermost area of the prostate that surrounds the urethra as it exits the bladder.

Transrectal ultrasound (TRUS) A scope is inserted though the rectum and produces an image of the prostate; urologists commonly use this procedure when doing a prostate biopsy.

Transurethral resection of the prostate (TURP) A surgical process to cut out tissue that is obstructing the urethra.

Tumour An abnormal lump of tissue that can be benign or cancerous.

TRUS *See* Transrectal ultrasound.

TURP *See* Transurethral resection of the prostate.

Ultrasound A diagnostic test that uses very high frequency sound waves to create an image of internal organs and structures, such as the prostate.

Ureters Two small tubes that carry urine from the kidneys to the bladder.

Urethra The tube through which urine and ejaculate leave the body.

Urethral stricture A narrowing of the urethra that blocks or decreases the flow of urine. Strictures are caused by scarring from a medical procedure or an injury.

Urgency A sudden need to urinate.

Urinary retention When the bladder has trouble emptying due to a blockage.

Urologist A surgeon who specializes in problems associated with the kidneys, ureters, bladder, prostate, urethra and testicles.

Vacuum constrictive device (VCD) A device that creates a vacuum around the penis to create an erection.

Vas deferens Two small, muscular tubes that carry sperm into the urethra.

VCD *See* Vacuum constrictive device.

Voiding Passing urine.

resources

Please note that these resources are included here for information only. Inclusion does not imply endorsement by the authors. Always talk to your doctor or nurse before changing any aspect of your treatment.

Prostate Cancer Information

Canadian Prostate Cancer Risk Calculator

A calculator provided by Sunnybrook Health Sciences Centre to evaluate prostate cancer risk using common risk factors.
http://www.prostaterisk.ca
http://www.sunnybrook.ca
/content/?page=3144

Canadian Urological Association

Patient information, news, and the latest urology research.
Email: cua@cua.org
http://www.cua.org
http://www.uroinfo.ca/

The Prostate Centre— Princess Margaret Hospital of the University Health Network (Canadian)

Patient information, the latest urology research, and publications.
http://www.prostatecentre.ca

American Urological Association (AUA) (US)

Patient information, the latest research, and publications.
1000 Corporate Boulevard
Linthicum, MD 21090, US
Tel: 410-689-3700
Fax: 410-689-3800
Email: aua@auanet.org
http://www.auanet.org

AUA Foundation: The Official Foundation of the American Urological Association (US)

Partners with healthcare professionals to provide information and resources to patients and their families on a range of urological conditions.
1000 Corporate Boulevard
Linthicum, MD 21090, US
Tel: 410-689-3700
Fax: 410- 689- 3998
Toll-free Urology Health Line: 1-800-828-7866
Email: auafoundation@auafoundation.org
http://www.urologyhealth.org/

National Cancer Institute at the National Institutes of Health (US)

Provides comprehensive information, resources, reference materials, with a live online chat feature. Services available in English and Spanish.
Toll-free information service:
1-800-4-CANCER (1-800-422-6237)
6116 Executive Boulevard
Suite 300
Bethesda, MD 20892-8322, US
http://www.cancer.gov/

Support Groups and Services

Prostate Cancer Canada

Public education, advocacy, research and support for patients and their families. Includes an online community for prostate cancer patients and their families with an email program that connects patient questions directly to doctors.
2 Lombard Street, 3rd Floor
Toronto, ON M5C 1M1
Tel: 416-441-2131
Toll-free: 1-888-255-0333
Fax: 416-441-2325
Email: info@prostatecancer.ca
http://www.prostatecancer.ca/

Prostate Cancer Canada Network (PCCN)

Trained volunteers offer support in person, on the telephone and through the Internet for those who are being treated for prostate cancer. PCCN raises public awareness through events and newsletters and provides one-to-one support. Larger cities may have support groups for gay men.
Email: info@prostatecancer.ca
http://www.prostatecancer.ca/pccn.aspx

Canadian Cancer Society
Cancer Connection

A free, confidential telephone support service that puts you in touch with cancer survivors. Available nationwide.
Tel: 1-888-939-3333 (For registered peer support members)
Toll-free: 1-800-263-6750 (Ontario and select other province)
Email: ccs@cancer.ca
http://www.cancer.ca
Cancerconnection.ca

Cancer connection also offers an online support community where you can chat with cancer survivors.

http://www.cancerconnection.ca

Wellspring (Canadian)

A cancer support organization for all cancer patients. Includes groups specifically for gay men and their partners.
http://www.wellspring.ca

Malecare (US)

Patient information, online support group with special programs for African-American men, men diagnosed under age 50, men experiencing erectile dysfunction and for gay men.
125 Second Avenue
New York, NY 10003, US
Tel: 212-673-4920
Email: info@malecare.org
http://malecare.org/

The National LGBT Cancer Project—Out With Cancer (US)

An online social networking site for gay men, bisexuals, transgenders and lesbians who have been diagnosed with cancer.
Email: info@lgbtcancer.org
http://lgbtcancer.org or http://www.outwithcancer.org

General Health Information

Canadian Centre for Activity and Aging (CCAA)

Community information, events, research and newsletters regarding aging.
Health Centre Annex, Lower Level, Suite 106
1490 Richmond Street London, ON N6G 2M3
Tel: 519-661-1603
Email: ccaa@uwo.ca
http://www.uwo.ca/actage

Health Canada

News, disease information and links.
http://www.hc-sc.gc.ca

267

Public Health Agency of Canada

General information about health for Canadians, including a section on heart health.
http://www.publichealth.gc.ca

Best Health Magazine (Canadian)

Online magazine providing health and wellness articles from a Canadian perspective
http://www.besthealthmag.ca

Telehealth Ontario (Canadian)

A 24-hours-a-day, 7-days-a-week hotline staffed by trained nurses with at least 5 years of experience.
Tel: 1-866-797-0000
http://www.health.gov.on.ca/en /public/programs/telehealth/

HealthFinder (US)

A service of the US Department of Health and Human Services that connects you to publications, non-profit organizations, databases, websites and support groups.
http://www.healthfinder.gov

WebMD (US)

Reliable health information including news, disease and drug information, health television guide, and tips for making a personal health plan and for searching the medical library.
http://www.webmd.com

Stress and Relaxation Information

Carleton University's Health and Counselling Services Resources (Canadian)

Links to stress information and self-tests.
http://www1.carleton.ca/health/

American Yoga Association (US)

General information on yoga, how to get started and how to choose a qualified yoga instructor.
Email: info@ americanyogaassociation.org
http://www.americanyogaassociation .org

Meditation Society of America (US)

Concepts and techniques of meditation plus suggested reading and online message board.
Email: medit8@meditationsociety.com
http://www.meditationsociety.com

Sam Houston State University Counseling Center (US)

Short relaxation techniques.
http://www.shsu.edu/~counsel/hs/shortrelax.html

The Transcendental Meditation Program (Canada/US)

Find out the benefits of, and how and where to learn, transcendental meditation.
Tel (US and Canada): 1-888-LEARN TM (1-888-532-7686)
http://www.maharishi.ca (Canada — French and English)
Email: questions@maharishi.ca
http://www.tm.org (US)

Nutrition and Fitness Information

Canadian Society for Exercise Physiology (CSEP)

The principal body for physical activity, health and fitness research and personal training in Canada. Provides links to resources, help with finding CSEP certified personal trainers, and physical activity guidelines.
Tel: 613-234-3755
Fax: 613- 234-3565
Toll-free: 1-877-651-3755
Email: info@csep.ca
http://www.csep.ca

Canadian Wellness

A directory of fitness, diet, health, nutrition, and other wellness-related professionals and their services.
Email: info@canadianwellness.com
http://www.canadianwellness.com

Dietitians of Canada

Nutrition resources and news.
Email: centralinfo@dieticians.ca
http://www.dietitians.ca

Health Canada's Food and Nutrition Resources

How to choose food by reading labels, *Canada's Food Guide* and research reports.
http://www.hc-sc.gc.ca/fn-an/index -eng.php

Academy of Nutrition and Dietetics (US)

Daily tips and features about nutrition.
http://www.eatright.org

Alternative Therapies Information

Holistic & Alternative Medicine (US)

Chat, read or ask about alternative therapies.
http://www.altmedweb.com

MedlinePlus (US)

Information on herbal remedies.
http://www.nlm.nih.gov/medlineplus /herbalmedicine.html

National Center for Complementary and Alternative Medicine (US)

An official source of information, including links to other sites, current research and scientific information.
Toll-free: 1-888-644-6226
International : 301-519-3153
Email: info@nccam.nih.gov
http://nccam.nih.gov/

Natural Solutions Magazine

Holistic and alternative approaches to health. What's new in alternative medicine.
http://www.naturalsolutionsmag .com

Books

Heber D, Fair WR and Ornish D. *Nutrition and Prostate Cancer. CaPCURE Nutrition Project Monograph*, 2nd edn. Santa Monica, CA: CaPCURE, 1998.

Perlman G, and Drescher J. (eds). *A Gay Man's Guide to Prostate Cancer*. Binghamton, NY: The Hawthorn Press Inc, 2005.

Trachtenberg J, Fleshner N, Currie K, Santa Mina D et al. *Challenging Prostate Cancer: Nutrition, Exercise and You.* 2007.

PDF downloadable through The Prostate Centre, Princess Margaret Hospital, University Health Network. http://www.prostatecentre. ca/downloads/Challenging%20 Prostrate%20Cancer%20PDF. pdf?seid=2051&mid=47

your diary

This section of the book is for you to keep track of your tests, procedures, appointments and important contact information as you navigate through your treatment and recovery.

Keeping good records is a great way to take control and stay organized. Having everything at your fingertips will reduce the anxiety of trying to remember your medical history as you move through your tests, treatments and follow-up.

KEY CONTACT INFORMATION

Family physician _____

_____

Phone number _____

_____

Fax number _____

_____

Email _____

_____

Urologist _____

Phone number _____

Fax number _____

Email _____

Primary nurse _____

Phone number _____

Fax number _____

Email _____

Hospital/clinic name _____

Phone number _____

Fax number _____

Email _____

TEST RESULTS

Date	PSA: result	Scans (e.g., CT, ultrasound): result	Place where test was done

APPOINTMENTS

Pre-operative assessment

Time _____

Hospital _____

Address _____

Room number _____

Checklist of what to bring to pre-operative assessment

- Health card _____
- Insurance information _____
- Medications _____
- Medical health reports if available _____
- Written questions_____

Surgery

Time _____

Hospital _____

Address _____

Room number _____

Post-op follow-up appointment

Time _____

Hospital _____

Address _____

Room number _____

CURRENT AND PAST MEDICATIONS

including complementary therapies and supplements

Drug name	Date began drug	Purpose of drug	Dosage	Side effects	Dosage instructions

QUESTIONS FOR THE DOCTOR

SYMPTOMS

Symptom	Date	Time	Cause	Severity on scale of 1 to 10 (1=mild, 10=severe)	Duration

TAKING CONTROL OF YOUR LIFE

Support group and counsellor contact information

Address	Phone	Fax	Email

My Lifestyle Goals:	Current Weight _____

NOTES

NOTES

NOTES

NOTES

Index

Page numbers in **bold** indicate illustrations.

A

abdominal ultrasound, 52

absorbent pads, 147

acetaminophen (Tylenol), 234, 238

acetylsalicylic acid (ASA), 105

active surveillance, for prostate cancer, 75–76

activities, following surgery, 141–143

See also exercise

acute urinary retention, 50, 64, 79

adenomas, 47

adjuvant treatments, 154–155

adrenaline, 54–55

adrenergics, 54

adult incontinence products, 147–148

Advil (ibuprofen), 105

aerobic exercise, 210

aggressiveness rating of tumors, 41–42

alfuzosin (Xatral), 56, 58, 236

Alka-Seltzer, 105

allergy medications, 54–55

alpha-blockers, 56, 57–58, 236

5-alpha-reductase, 24

5-alpha-reductase inhibitors, 56–59, 236

alprostadil (MUSE, Caverject), 193–194, 196, 238

ALYX, 110

American Society of Clinical Oncology, 33

American Urological Association (AUA) symptom score, 52

anal sex, 220–222

androgen deprivation therapy. *See* antiandrogens; LHRH agonists; LHRH antagonists

androgens. *See* testosterone

anemia

caused by surgery, 109

reducing transfusion risk, 111–112

therapy, 237

treatments, 110, 231

285

M

male partners. *See* gay men

malignant hyperthermia, 104

man who has sex with men (MSM), 224
  See also gay men

massage, 168

Mayo Clinic, 155

meat, 20–21

medical students, 248

medication
  following surgery, 234–235
  for incontinence, 148
  for post-surgery pain, 132–134
  pre-surgery disclosure, 104, 105
  for prostate cancer prevention, 24–25
  side effects, 236–239
  before surgery, 231–232
  during surgery, 233
  See also drug therapy

meditation, 167

men (male partners). *See* gay men

metastatic prostate cancer
  drug therapy, 92–95, 154–155
  incidence of, 7
  pathology reports, 152
  positive margins, **153**
  tests for, 44–45

midazolam (Versed), 237

Midol, 105

morphine, 133, 234, 238

motivation to exercise, 214–215

MRI (magnetic resonance imaging), 45

MRI targeted focal therapy, 244

MRSA (methicillin-resistant *Staphylcoccus aureus*), 103–104

MSM (man who has sex with men), 224
  See also gay men

muscle relaxation, 167

MUSE (alprostadil), 193, 194, 196, 238

N

naproxen, 105

narcotics, 133, 134, 234, 238

nasal prongs, 131

National Cancer Institute (US), 12, 17, 34, 242

nausea, 234

negative margins, **153**

nerve grafting, 87

nerves
  damage to, 182, 183
  pudendal (erection), **6**
  sensory, 176, 198

nerve-sparing techniques, 87

New England Journal of Medicine, 24, 60, 86, 177

T

tadalafil (Cialis), 190–191, 196, 238

tamsulosin (Flomax), 56, 58, 236

Taxotere (docetaxel), 95, 231, 236

tea, 17–18

temporary-seed brachytherapy, 81, 82–83

terazosin (Hytrin), 58, 236

testes (testicles)
location of, **6**
in sexual activity, 178

testosterone
effect of drug therapy, 93–94, 231
effect on prostate cancer, 92–93
prostate enlargement and, 51

tests
for cancer spreading, 44–45
pre-surgery, 104
for prostate cancer, 29–34, 36–38

thighs, pain, swelling, redness, 117

three-dimensional conformal radiotherapy (3D-CRT), 80

thrombosis, 115, 117, 135

TNM staging system, 42–44

tolterodine (Detrol), 58, 133, 148, 234, 235, 237, 238

tomatoes, 14–15

Toradol (ketorolac), 133, 234, 238

transgender male to female, 225
See also gay men

transrectal ultrasound (TRUS)-guided biopsies, 36–40

transurethral microwave thermotherapy (TUMT), 66–67

transurethral resection of the prostate. *See* TURP

transversus abdominal plane (TAP) blocks, 133

treatment for prostate cancer
active surveillance, 75–77
choosing method, 97
clinical trials, 241–242
new advances in, 242–244
watchful waiting, 74–75, 76–77
See also drug therapy; radical prostatectomy; radiotherapy

Trelstar (leuprolide), 93, 236

TRUS (transrectal ultrasound)-guided biopsies, 36–40

tumors
aggressiveness of, 41–42, 73
spread of, 42–44
tests for spread of, 44–45

TUMT (transurethral microwave thermotherapy), 66–67
TURP (transurethral resection of the prostate)
  determining success of, 67
  procedure, 60–62, **63**
  pros and cons, 63–66, 69
two-spirited men. *See* gay men
Tylenol (acetaminophen), 234, 238

U

ultrasound
  for biopsies, 36–40
  for BPH diagnosis, 52
  new treatments for cancer, 242–243
underwear for incontinence, 147
University of Chicago, 177
University of Toronto, 170
ureters
  function of, 3
  injury in surgery, 149–150
  location of, **4**
urethra
  location of, **4**, **6**
  normal function, 4
urethral clamps, 148
urethral stricture, 53, 145
urethral suppositories, 194
urethrotomy, 145

urge incontinence, 65, 146
urinary incontinence.
  See incontinence
urinary retention, 50, 64, 79
urination
  changes in voiding, 28, 49–50
  difficulties following surgery, 145
  difficulty in, 47
  following catheter removal, 145
  nerve sparing in surgery, 87
  normal function, 3–5
  See also incontinence
urine tests for prostate cancer, 36
uroflow test, 52
urologists, 86
US Census, 223–224
US Centers for Disease Control and Prevention, 222
US Department of Health and Human Services, 20
US Food and Drug Administration (FDA), 25, 243
US National Cancer Institute, 12, 17, 34, 242
US Preventative Services Task Force (USPSTF), 32

V

vacuum constrictive devices (VCDs), 194–195, 196
vardenafil (Levitra, Staxyn), 190–192, 196, 238
vas deferens
function of, 179
location of, 5, **6**
vasectomies, 10
VCDs (vacuum constrictive devices), 194–195, 196
vegetarians, 21
verbal consent, 107
Versed (midazolam), 237
Viagra (sildenafil), 189–191, 196, 238
visualization, 167–168
vitamin D, 18–19
vitamin E, 16–17, 60, 105
volunteers, 250
vomiting, 234
VRE (vancomycin-resistant *Enterococcus*), 103–104

W

walking, 142, 169
warfarin (Coumadin), 237
watchful waiting
for BPH (benign prostatic hyperplasia), 53–55, 68
for prostate cancer, 74–75, 76–77, 95
water pills, 55
weight loss, 170
wine, 17–18
women, sexual experience for, 187–188
work, following surgery, 143
wound care, 138–139
written consent, 107

X

Xatral (alfuzosin), 56, 58, 236

Z

zinc, 20
Zoladex (goserelin), 93, 236